GET WELL—EVEN
IN TODAY'S CONFUSION,
UNCERTAINTY, AND FEAR

To Mr Jude —
Thank you for welcoming
a different point of view
on your wonderful Podcast!
Loved meeting you,

Sandy

GET WELL—EVEN IN TODAY'S CONFUSION, UNCERTAINTY, AND FEAR

SANDY COWEN

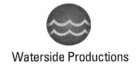

Waterside Productions

Cover design by Scott Anderson

ISBN-13: 978-1-958848-74-6 print edition
ISBN-13: 978-1-958848-75-3 e-book edition

Waterside Productions
2055 Oxford Ave
Cardiff, CA 92007
www.waterside.com

This book is dedicated to the healing warriors who've decided to fight for their health!

TABLE OF CONTENTS

INTRODUCTION

In 2008 my first book was published titled *Get Well: Even When You've Been Told You Can't*. That book was the first of its kind as a holistic healing handbook of sorts that managed the expectations for anyone wanting to venture out into the world of alternative options. It was a process book, not a prescriptive one, and was written primarily for people facing serious chronic illness as well as life-threatening diseases. The book provided practical explanations about how mind-body-spirit medicine works, shared a little about my personal health history prior to 2010, and walked people step-by-step through a holistic healing journey.

So, at first, I thought I'd update that book to include my last healing journey, from 2009 through 2017, and make more current the research points that were now outdated. The content was solid and could still serve as the empowerment tool people still needed to take control of their health and healing. Then, I said, *nope—the recent pandemic has caused so much change in the world and not for the better. I'm afraid people today need messages even more empowering.*

The way the COVID-19 pandemic was managed chipped away at the confidence many people had in the federal medical institutions that control our health care system. The remainder of the population remained fear-ridden and obediently followed whatever order was being handed out with some still wearing masks and others lining up for one booster after another.

The fear-based reaction people still had flew in the face of quotes from the Centers for Disease Control and Prevention (CDC), which said, "Well, we may have gotten it wrong." And others in institutional medical leadership either backpedaled with the release of new data and test results or jumped ship. At this point, I believe the public is wary and still fearful of what lurks around the corner in terms of future threats to their health. Fear is no place to reside.

With that said, this book is designed to help reinstate trust, although not to the source you'd expect. It will educate and inspire individuals to feel more empowered and in control of their own health. It will also help mitigate the fear that has spread relentlessly and is still encouraged after nearly three years.

Now that I've said that, let me explain my qualifications to write this book. If you're a new reader or someone unaware of my background—I have an impressive track record (over many decades) of completely recovering from a rash of chronic and life-threatening conditions without the help of conventional medicine or pharmaceutical drugs. The conditions included rheumatoid arthritis, leukemia (twice), hyperthyroidism (Graves' disease), chronic allergies, psoriasis, and finally neutropenia. Again, using only natural methods, I have survived and continue to thrive.

It's important to note that I'm not against conventional medicine since I use that form of care for diagnoses and a few other reasons. I've just learned to not overuse it—especially the pharmaceuticals. This book will help readers see the logic behind my shift since so many surprising facts are revealed in this book. One being that Americans today are overprescribed medicines and is one of the causes for our society becoming much less healthy overall.

So, as you read on, I'll shine a light on why the transformation of scientific, conventional medicine in the last few decades may not have served its patients well and what we can learn from the last three years of the COVID-19 crisis. Readers might also find that being more discriminating in health decisions is prudent; a more inclusive approach to health care is often warranted, and questioning is a patient's right. I do not encourage readers to leave the world of conventional medicine, I just present information that will help them become more open to other possibilities and more educated about when to use each.

I hope each of you will approach this book with an open mind and become, if nothing else, curious about how a woman nearly eighty years old managed to waltz through the landmines of disease and illness since the early 1980s to find a new and extraordinary quality of life as the years continued. How she sailed through the coronavirus scare is fascinating as well. A healthy body, even if it once wasn't, makes many things possible. Healing, you know, isn't a destination; it's a process.

You might also learn how to adjust your thinking, suspend judgment more often, trust your body more, and recognize the power of your miraculous immune system. You'll discover how mind-body-sprit medicine (holistic healing) works and be able to apply it to your life to heal on many more levels than the obvious. In doing so, you might also find a healthy life, total peace, and so much joy each day that you may feel compelled to share it with others.

In today's very confusing, uncertain, and fear-based world, it's time for a little hope, healthy reflection, and inspiration. This book promises to present many holistic approaches to healing that are harmless and improve the possibility for people to overcome chronic conditions, auto-immune and immunodeficiency diseases, and even viruses!

Welcome to new possibilities!

Chapter 1

AND THEN THE LIGHT CAME ON

After a traumatic period in American history brought on by the nearly three-year pandemic, a tiny light appeared at the end of the tunnel. It wasn't the end of the coronavirus pandemic—since we'll all be living with one virus or another forever—it was something else.

There was a short flash of information that surfaced toward the end of the mandates, restrictions, and recommendations that opened the door to individual empowerment and more personal freedom for everyone! That little flash was brief, and I guess subtle, but I certainly noticed it. This is how it began.

One day, very early in the crisis, a YouTube video appeared with a doctor talking about a supplement that could help the immune system. Then another video by Dr. Oz appeared, and shortly after, an internet article was posted that was quickly removed about early therapeutics that were working. What was valuable about that last article was the ingredients of that healing cocktail—one being the mineral zinc.

What followed was a whack-a-mole experience—with a voice from over there and another from way out there popping up to mention supplements, specifically vitamins and one mineral that might help the body fight against viruses. Those messages came and went so quickly most didn't catch them. Those who did may not have understood their significance at the time.

Then President Trump developed COVID-19, and when he was recounting the ingredients in the therapeutic cocktail he was given by the White House physician to help him quickly recover, he mentioned that zinc was part of that cocktail mix. If you recall, the media and medical "experts" assigned to guide us through the pandemic response all ridiculed the core therapeutic and totally ignored the zinc comment. The media, of course, followed suit.

Now, fast forward six months. After thousands of Americans had already died, the public began to hear and suddenly some of the medical leadership began acknowledging that vitamin D and zinc existed. These were still always random comments, and the first came from clinical physicians appearing on television. For the first time these voices weren't canceled or discredited. The context in which either vitamin D or zinc were mentioned had to do with the power both had to boost our immunity to help prevent or recover more quickly from the coronavirus. A miracle, I thought—not the information, which I'd known for decades, but that the words immune system and a couple supplements were being mentioned at all.

I was thrilled because I had been taking both those supplements for years for my immune system issues, along with healthy doses of vitamin C and some magnesium to help the vitamin D absorption, and I had a long history of recovery. Most other folks were isolated in the world of conventional medicine—where vitamins and minerals were basically ignored. The mass population had no idea that there were simple, harmless, and affordable supplements that could be bought at their local natural market or health food stores to help keep them healthy. They still wouldn't have known except that everyone's eyes, including theirs, had been riveted on their televisions watching the play-by-play of how quickly this virus was spreading.

Although I'd love to give credit to scientific medicine for finally acknowledging this fact, it didn't come from the medical leadership in Washington, DC. It came first from regular frontline doctors who had been treating patients throughout the crisis and knew what worked, on a practical sense, and what didn't. Those frontline doctors, or clinical physicians, didn't have a voice in the policy surrounding COVID-19's management. No, that was all in the hands of the academics, administrators, and researchers at the bureaucratic medical institutional level who were calling the shots. They were the designated "experts."

Because of the qualifications of those leading the pandemic response, I was always skeptical about the management of this effort. The more I watched, the more I became certain as the lives of Americans were needlessly compromised and, in some cases, ruined by the mandates, regulations, and recommendations being doled out from the podiums. Had immune system education been brought to the forefront earlier to help the public shore up their defenses, the country may have prevented the devastating effects of this one specific virus.

Instead, the focus was on what scientific medicine was going to do to help us—not what we could do to help ourselves. We were given behavioral mandates like when to put on and take off our masks; how to stand six feet away, where the floor markers required; and to absolutely stay as far away from our elderly friends and family as possible regardless of if they needed us or not. In fact, it was best if we just isolated and stayed at home.

All the while, while the public dutifully obeyed, the numerous podcasts and YouTube videos about the immune system, vitamin D deficiency, and zinc began were randomly appearing. The first ones as early as March 9, 2020. Even Dr. Oz's video appeared on April 10, 2020, advocating for zinc and existing therapeutics as a likely remedy. No one seemed to notice because everyone, in panic mode, stayed fixated on television news.

It took many more months for the medical experts who were setting policy from a national perspective to get on board. Pretty soon an article that reinforced zinc as possibly effective against the coronavirus appeared in September 2020 on WebMD. Countless other studies on the subject in medical journals and online resources prior, well before that, that in retrospect now couldn't be ignored. So, vitamin D was adopted as helpful early into 2021 without too much resistance. A year after the coronavirus threat appeared.

One such article was titled "Demographic differences and trends of vitamin D insufficiency in the US population, 1988–2004," which came from the National Institutes of Health (NIH), *National Library of Medicine* and appeared on pubmed.ncbi.nim.nih.gov. I'd like to quote it directly. The abstract of the article says this: "Vitamin D insufficiency is associated with suboptimal health. The prevalence of vitamin D insufficiency may be rising, but population-based trends are uncertain. We sought to evaluate US population trends in vitamin D insufficiency." (1)

They go on to explain their methods and statistical results, but I want to jump right to their conclusions. "National data demonstrate a marked decrease in serum 25 (OH)D levels from the 1988–1994 to the 2001–2004 NHANES data collections. Racial/ethnic differences have persisted and may have important implications for known health disparities. Current recommendations for vitamin D supplantation are inadequate to address the growing epidemic of vitamin D insufficiency." Translation? A decrease in vitamin D levels has been occurring since 1988 and is connected to health issues. Current recommended vitamin D levels are inadequate to address the growing epidemic of this insufficiency. In other words, therapeutic doses are needed to curb the decline.

If you do your own research, you will see that the vitamin D insufficiency levels have continued to get worse worldwide, and the problem has been known to the medical establishment since 2004 with the results frequently published—yet the agencies responsible for patient safety in the United States didn't notice. Therefore, they did nothing to notify the public, encourage our doctors to inform their patients, or recommend testing.

Similarly ignored were study after study acknowledging the efficacy of zinc against viruses appearing in various articles to which everyone had access. One such article within the very same pubmed.gov source as mentioned above was titled: "The Role of Zinc in Antiviral Immunity—PubMed," which states in its abstract that "Zinc is an essential trace element that is crucial for growth, development, and the maintenance of immune function." (2)

Other articles were also all over the internet addressing the value of zinc against the common cold virus, which is in the coronavirus family, and how zinc inhibits viral replication. Even one medical article talks about zinc helping dimmish the extent of COVID-19, not as a silver bullet, but as a worthy contributor to combating the infection.

Still, for some unearthly reason, scientific-based conventional medicine continued to distinguish the common cold virus from the COVID-19 virus although they are both exist within the coronavirus family. Hello—the immune system doesn't care what name you slap on the virus or what strain it is. To the immune system a virus is a virus is a virus. This magnificent system is designed to fight any foreign invader, including viruses, bacteria, parasites, and even cancers. It doesn't distinguish one from another. Besides, supplements designed to strengthen the immune system are there to strengthen our immunity, not to kill the viruses themselves. The immune system, when healthy, does all the killing.

The one exception to supplements that primarily strengthen us is zinc, which also does kill many viruses with immediate contact. Anyway, too much detail for this chapter, so just bear with me until we progress further into the book.

In upcoming chapters, we'll learn more about our immune systems, what we can do to keep them healthy, how we compromise our immune health, and other facts relative to empowerment that lay outside the world of conventional medicine.

Again, I can't say often enough what a blessing it was to see the topic of our immune systems popping up in conversation as the COVID-19 pandemic evolved. Once there is awareness, there can be further education as curiosity hopefully takes over and people begin to ask, *are there really things I can do to help myself*?

Should we be critical of doctor for not educating us about prevention?

I don't think we can blame conventional medicine for not being on top of what patients can really do to help themselves because preventive medicine just isn't in their wheelhouse. They're taught to treat what the patient presents at the time of a visit, not educate patients on how to stay healthy. The presenting issue comes first, and that's really all physicians have time for. Neither empowering their patients in prevention nor being well informed about remedies and therapies available in the natural world were ever part of the medical school curriculum. A good reminder that our medical doctors don't know everything about everything.

As will be documented as we proceed, if you want to know more about surgery, drugs and pharmaceuticals, radiation, and related therapies—ask a medical doctor. If you want to know more about how your lifestyle choices, what you eat, and how you think might matter in your health and healing—ask other providers.

Medical doctors are also not responsible for how pharmaceuticals have dominated their treatment model—nor do they have responsibility for the extraordinary influence Big Pharma has in all facets of medical, educational, and conventional medicine's regulatory world.

Remember, the pharmaceutical industry is exactly that—an industry. They're in business to make money, which isn't a bad thing, it's just a thing. So, pharmaceutical companies will only develop products on which they can hold patents and increase revenues. Nobody can hold a patent on vitamins and minerals or the natural herbs that are found throughout nature. With no perceived profitability, there's no interest in touching that marketplace. Everything pharmaceutical companies deal with is man-made, chemically based, or chemically influenced and on which patents can be acquired.

Nobody is to blame for not teaching us how to take care of ourselves; that's really an individual's responsibility and for family and friends to help. Also, once a person becomes more aware, they can reach out to providers like osteopaths (DOs), who also have a medical license but also possess skeletal training; naturopaths; homeopaths; holistic MDs who lead with natural methods and prefer drugs as a last resort. Such MDs aren't available in all cities, but there are other alternative medical providers who could fill that gap.

Remember, scientific medicine has only been around in the form we know it today since the 1920s, even though the first peer-reviewed medical information was published in the late 1800s. So, medical physicians focus on the advances made over the last two centuries, not in the centuries that came before, and certainly not those (although currently being used) dating back two to five thousand years.

Final point, just because conventional medical doctors don't help patients understand the importance of a healthy immune system doesn't mean science ignores the subject. Science does study the immune system but primarily to find out how they can stimulate it with drug therapy, replicate parts of it eventually, or render other parts inactive to stop an autoimmune response. Conventional medicine is focused on how to fix the immune system externally instead of how to strengthen it internally.

Why my story is unique.

Over the last forty years, even though I was previously only exposed to conventional medicine in my lifetime, by the time I reached my late thirties, I became so discouraged with my health and the limited ability of my doctors that I walked away. It's amazing how quicky being pushed into the pool can teach a person to swim!

In the process, I learned to keep a very faulty immune system in check and totally recover from a host of autoimmune and immune deficiency diseases—all naturally and without doing any harm to my body in the process.

So, my life serves as an example of how miraculously even a faulty immune system can recover and how a person can grow smarter with each disease—to eventually learn the tools they need to use to recover multiple times but remain healthier at the end. Ironic since through those subsequent decades, I wasn't getting any younger.

I learned about personal responsibility by default and how most of us contribute to the state of our health. I learned that even with a family gene history that's negative, vulnerability won't manifest in our lifetime if we learn how prevent what we're most likely to contract.

As you read on, I hope you'll become more empowered, too, and realize how the magnificent machine you were given at birth and its extraordinary immune system work continually on your behalf to dodge the bullets from autoimmunity, immune deficiency, and even bacteria, viruses, and cancer. Not everyone will fully recover from whatever they have, and not everyone will prevent future disease, because that takes discipline, commitment, and patience, but it is possible to improve any condition, even in the short term—enough to delight your doctor and reduce the strengths of some of the medications you're taking.

Why is COVID-19 and the subject of viruses an early focus in this book?

Because viruses are a fact of life, they've been with us for a long time, and don't appear to be going away anytime soon—we need to understand them more and be terrified less. We also need to realize that it's impossible to create enough vaccines to stop everything because viruses morph and change so rapidly that whatever worked months prior can be useless today. So, we'd better become smarter as a population and learn how we can protect ourselves from one of the realities of life—not merely wait for science to try playing catch-up.

In fact, I'll bet readers, who've survived the last three years of uncertainty and confusion, are left somewhat dazed and even fearful of what might lurk just around the corner. At this point having trust issues and becoming more skeptical makes perfect sense.

So, consider this book a giant flashlight focused backward initially to help reveal additional information that might have been obscured in darkness or even hidden intentionally. Hindsight is always helpful, and light itself has a wonderful way of empowering those with their eyes wide open.

Chapter 2

20/20 HINDSIGHT

A review of what happened over the last three years might be in order since long after the pandemic was declared over, people are still walking around with masks on. Of course, that might be because of the CDC's continual and conflicting recommendations, which we'll also scrutinize in a bit.

Let's begin from when the pandemic was declared in the spring of 2020. We knew a virus had entered our country from some unknown origin. We also knew that this virus seemed to be spreading quickly and nobody knew how deadly it was—or if it was deadly at all. The experts who were in charge were the people we looked up to and trusted. Everyone—the public, the politicians, and the media—believed what they said. The organizations in charge were based in Washington, DC and bear the responsibility for the initial mandates and policy recommendations that were set forth. None of those edicts, by the way, were flexible, and all were presented as absolutely the only option because they were based on "science." It's hard to forget that word because we were reminded of it, ad nauseum, over the ensuing two-plus years.

The experts from Washington, DC were the primary messengers regarding the coronavirus, specifically COVID-19, as it was called. They represented the CDC, the NIH, the Food and Drug Administration (FDA) and the National Institute of Allergy and Infectious Diseases (NIAID), as well as the individual who led and coordinated the White House Coronavirus Response Team (2020). Each played a role, the most visible being Dr. Anthony Fauci, who also happened to have been, and still is as of the writing of this book, the highest-paid bureaucrat in all of government. In a less visible role but also players behind the scenes were the leadership of the FDA and the American Medical Association (AMA), which supported all efforts to their membership. Let's not forget the World Health Organization (WHO), a United Nations agency whose responsibility it has been to promote health and help keep the world safe. That organization was hovering in the background too. Yet, from the beginning, the WHO's tight relationship with the Chinese Communist Party, their true agenda, and their actual loyalty to the citizens of the world they swore to protect some question. Regardless, the WHO held notable influence over our government agencies.

As the most visible spokesperson, Dr. Anthony Fauci ended up being the authority and the ultimate voice about COVID-19 representing government and science. Throughout the first two-and-a-half years, the media didn't let us forget how important Dr. Fauci was, not for a moment. That is until he announced his retirement in the fall of 2022, just before the 2022 midterm elections. More about that later.

How did government determine what to do?

Now, this is where my confusion escalated since the public will never know exactly how the sausage is made within the hallowed halls of the federal government, but we can assess the methodology of the rollout and execution we did observe. In a nutshell, what I saw didn't fit into any model I'd ever seen before for executing any type of effective plan.

Normally, when a plan is formulated for something as huge as this, the smartest gather to precisely identify the problem, then brainstorm to find solutions that might work—analyzing the short-term and long-term effects or risks versus rewards of each and finally pick the best solution to implement. That one solution might end up being a simple fix or involve a comprehensive approach, but accompanying that solution is generally some overall strategy with the desired outcome clearly articulated. *Slow the curve* comes to mind. After that, I didn't hear a particular deliverable communicated to the public, nor did I see any periodic review and modification of the original strategy, nor did I see any adjustments to the execution plan being made along the way.

Once the CDC and other medical leaders set the policy, they dug in whenever a logical question was raised by the public, the media, or other medical professionals about their process or the results. Eventually, we were all trained to stop asking any more questions. Even when the White House, in the beginning, put pressure on the medical team to limit the lockdowns to mitigate collateral damage, the experts in charge didn't budge. Everything they said was based on science, and that was that.

Now, you might be thinking that in science the problem-solving process might be different. Such differences are mainly in the vocabulary used and the length of time it takes to begin any rollout phase. First, scientists must have proof that a strategy will work, and proving anything through the scientific method takes years.

For something to be scientifically proven, the initial stage is merely a hypothesis. This is how a hypothesis is reached. First, they consider the question, begin the research process, develop hypotheses—generally multiple ones, and run experiments and testing while analyzing the data. Throughout the process ideas are rejected or accepted and the methodology is tweaked until the conclusions are reached at the end. The end generally takes many years. Science itself is ever changing since even a hypothesis most agreed upon initially can later be proven wrong.

This doesn't sound remotely like what happened in the case of the COVID-19 issue. In that situation, everything was driven by the government's academic, administrative, bureaucratic, and research-based theory with little or no input from frontline doctors in the field who were treating patients already infected—some very effectively. Although the in-field testing data provided some anecdotal evidence, that was immediately dismissed by those in charge.

This all begs the question why the rush for only science to provide answers, why weren't modifications made along the way, and what was the real agenda? We're left wondering.

The first inconsistency—the masking.

The initial confusion began with the masks. Regardless of the reason, people were told masks were useless, then we were specifically asked to wear them, and then mandated to do so. At one point, wearing multiple masks at a time was encouraged! At each stage, Dr. Fauci was unwavering in his directives, and other leaders followed along compliantly. Each time, Fauci insisted the conclusion was based on science. The media went along, never questioning but just nodding and repeating, which made thinking individuals scratch their heads.

After a person hears the "based on science" comment over and over—even while the instructions keep changing—intelligent human beings notice the disconnects. In addition, the rest of medical leadership's lame efforts to reinforce Fauci's and the CDC's guidelines began to ring hollow.

Americans are a generous bunch and seem to give their leaders the benefit of the doubt. *Well, the science may have changed*, some may have thought. *Maybe they kept learning more as time went on*, others may have felt. I almost bought in to that rationale since there was some logic to the argument, but when statistics from other parts of the world began surfacing that revealed that masks and strict lockdowns weren't preventing the spread of COVID-19 at all, more questions for me and from others arose.

All the while, the media, politicians, and medical experts were parading around with some wearing scarf-type masks that pulled up over their mouth and nose—some made from colorful cloth—with others wearing paper masks, but very few wore the N95 or KN95 masks, which are tighter-fitting and more effective. Anyway, masks were all over the place in terms of what they looked like and how people wore them. Even when masks were required in stores, people wandered around indoors with their noses exposed and masks barely covering their mouths. For nearly a year, nobody said a thing.

There are photos of Dr. Anthony Fauci, physician, scientist, immunologist, and director of NIAID in paper masks. Dr. Deborah Birx, physician and diplomat who served as the White House Coronavirus Response Coordinator under President Trump from 2020–2021, who specialized in immunology, vaccine research, and global health also wore paper surgical masks. It was February 2022 before the government began issuing free N95 masks to the public, two full years after this pandemic occurred. Regardless of shortage issues, which were never announced, these were apparent inconsistencies that made the public question whether these people knew what they were talking about or not.

Clinical physicians in the field were taking a different position on masks, but their voices were muted, discredited, or they were canceled on social media and banned from mass media appearances. Mask wearing by young children is still fiercely debated by people who recognize the damage it can and did cause to early socialization and learning.

Even in mid-2022, information remained inconsistent. Although a federal judge on April 18, 2022, struck down the federal government's nationwide mask order for public transit, commercial flights, and transportation hubs such as airports and train stations as being unlawful, and the US Transportation Security Administration stopped enforcing that mandate for major airlines, (3) the CDC didn't seem to care. Immediately after—on May 3, 2022, it reissued the recommendation that people ages two and older wear masks while on public transportation and at transportation hubs. (4)

As of August 2022, although 98 percent of the K-12 schools in the United States no longer required masks, the CDC, in its guidance for schools, still recommended universal indoor masking in K-12 schools and early education programs that are in counties with a high COVID-19 community level. (5) That gave enormous power to the school board leadership to interpret what the community level threat was and whether to consider a recommendation from the CDC as a requirement or not. All of this was needlessly confusing to many. To others, still gripped by fear, we saw adults continuing to walk around nearly empty stores or outside in masks two-and-a-half years later, when the pandemic threat had long since passed.

There were other inconsistencies too.

There were other issues throughout those three years that caused jaws to drop as well—including lockdowns, school closures, the restriction of early therapeutics, and the overreaching mandates that stripped people of their personal freedom. Each of these restrictive policies were rolled out with inconsistencies in the approach, the timing, and by geographic location.

Everything was subject to reporting the spread rate—whether data was accurate or not—and not the lethal nature of the virus if that was even the case. In retrospect, much of the reporting proved incomplete or inaccurate.

No debates occurred in a public forum. It was always a mandate here and a random "out in the wilderness" voice there. The consistency always came from the institutional medical bureaucrats and media who were in control and in lockstep with their "scientific" interpretation of the facts. The resulting collateral damage that occurred was ignored.

Everybody else, regardless of their individual credibility or professional platform, who spoke up with a differing opinion or questions were treated like isolated malcontents. The heck with the opinions of physicians who were treating patients and the heck with experts in diverse fields who understood the psychological impact of some of the mandates. The heck with anybody who had a differing opinion, this was science, *man!*

Over the first twenty-four months, you'd have thought the media would ask more questions for further clarity—but they didn't. They picked their side early, and all other opinions were shut down. Authoritarian-style censorship always causes a reaction with the public, whether it is openly voiced or not. Such action also breeds increased skepticism.

All anyone ever talked about was how much COVID was spreading, not how deadly it was or wasn't or who seemed to suffer the most. There was a broad brush used to paint the threat as overarching, so the fear kept growing because people believed everybody was at risk. In the end, immeasurable harm resulted for our children, our elders, small businesses, and the overall economy, and this overreach may have created the impetus for increased cases of drug additions and suicides that followed.

All this could have been prevented had we asked questions earlier and had answers followed. Instead, we faced a steady stream of doublespeak and the obfuscation of facts. The result is that I, for one, became more even more suspicious of scientific, conventional medicine and its real agenda.

Why was the focus on the spread instead of the death rate?

We can only assume. When the public is afraid, they're easier to control, they look to someone in authority for answers, and the tendency is to believe whatever they're told. In the case of COVID-19, even though the messaging was inconsistent at best, people still believed the authorities. Even so, the fear spreading continued.

By focusing on the wrong thing, medical leadership, politicians, and leadership promulgated more and more fear. With a rapidly spreading virus and that being the only focus—the public began to dread the spread instead of asking about the seriousness of the disease. The coverage was ten parts spread and one part dead.

When deaths were discussed, no one drilled down on the reasons for a patient's rapid decline after being admitted to the hospital. If one entered the hospital with COVID-19, it was believed to be a death sentence. Yet, there could have been lots of reasons for the multiple deaths in that environment. Was it because patients were encouraged to wait too long to seek help? Was it because physicians were disallowed from prescribing common therapeutics others used? Or was it the extreme seriousness of the disease itself? Could it have been the hospital's treatment protocol that was at fault? Or the lack of early treatment that was the cause? Or was it totally due to comorbidity issues? Nobody told us and there was no reliable data available so we could draw our own conclusions.

The initial strategy seemed to be to spread as much fear throughout the population as possible, causing people to isolate, businesses to close, and everybody to freeze while the medical establishment figured out what to do next. The fact that they didn't know what to do is not a sin, the fact that they terrified the public to do nothing themselves while they waited for a silver bullet (the vaccines) was a sin, in my opinion.

Left to our own devices, you'd be surprised how quickly word-of-mouth answers would have spread and frontline doctors, who were getting results, could help so many more. Instead, the strategy of these leaders was absolute and ended up resulting in countless other consequences we have yet to quantify.

The biggest question for me throughout was where was the comprehensive and meaningful data? We'd hear reports about where in the country outbreaks were occurring and which races or ethnic groups were most affected, but there was little or no ongoing data focusing on how many died from the disease and what were the ages of those fatalities.

Now that such data is finally available, it might be fascinating to look.

How many died from COVID-19 and how old were they?

The age-defined statistics took forever to surface in a pure form without emphasis on the racial or geographic subsets. These figures appeared to be the most comprehensive and current at the time of this writing. They were obtained by statista.com and include all deaths in the United States from January 2020 through October 5, 2022.

Of the 1,056,002 total deaths, 549,121 (52%) were from the population 75 years or older.

Those aged 65–74 realized 242,880 deaths (23%), and people in the 50–64 age group counted for 190,080 fatalities (18%).

That means 93% of *all* deaths were people over 50 years of age, and we might assume that those 50–64 were likely suffering from one or more of the comorbidity issues. Anyone from 18–49 only accounted for 7% of the deaths. The numbers under 18 were so small, they were statistically irrelevant. (6)

This alone begs the question of why vaccines were mandated for everyone? Why were lockdowns and masks mandated for everyone? Why wasn't the bulk of the prevention focused on those at high-risk and the elderly?

Why didn't we adopt more targeted policies to help the most vulnerable?

Anybody with a lick of sense would have figured out that the most vulnerable among us would be individuals with compromising health conditions and the very elderly—maybe even small children. The early facts would have easily confirmed the first two groups and small children would have been immediately discounted since their risk was so low. Instead, we waited for reporting that never came.

The institutional medical community does deserve a little credit for identifying early on the comorbidity issues such as obesity, diabetes, cardiovascular disease, and individuals who were incapable of developing a normal immune response—in other words the immunocompromised—as well as the very elderly. Still, the government didn't really act on that information to develop targeted strategies for each population segment or even for that group en masse. Instead, they just told us all to stay away and protect the elderly at all costs.

Elderly individuals were isolated in nursing homes, even when they were dying, and their loved ones were restricted from visits. We were also told to don masks so, by accident, we didn't cause another's death by standing too close in a public arena or even outside. The warnings went on for many, many months with the initial focus being for the total public to obey. Guilt was used to accompany the mandates, and the directives were also phrased in a way that anyone who questioned compliance was attempting to kill Aunt Martha or their grandmothers. Finally, the restrictions grew and grew until people began judging each other. Fear fueled judgment and turned elements of the population against each other.

People who realized they were in the high-risk group, not necessarily the aging population, were so terrified that many stayed in their homes with limited public access for two years. I happen to know a couple of them.

A state of emergency was declared by our government leaders, but that emergency crisis was being applied to everyone, not simply those at risk.

A closer look at the nature of viruses.

When I heard a vaccine was on the horizon for a virus, more than one red flag went up. I happen to understand how viruses operate, having been very vulnerable to them my entire adult life, and having survived them all.

COVID-19, as you know, is a virus, and viruses are very tricky to vaccinate against. That's why year after year science tries to get the flu vaccine right—yes, flu is a virus too. Some years they do a little better than others. The reason is because it's hard to predict the strain that might surface. Viruses, as we remember, are unpredictable and morph again and again like the flu viruses do. It's not only the way they transform themselves, but also the way they develop resistance to many antiviral drugs thrown at them, so it takes stronger and stronger drugs or different drugs to be effective.

Although viruses are a fact of life, the good news is that although most viruses frequently spread easily, very few of them kill the healthy among us.

So, why did *this* virus kill so many more people? Was it because the virus was that lethal? Or was it because our population had become less healthy over the years? Think about the possibility of that last option for a moment.

Is our nation healthy enough to withstand viral pandemics?

Our society is not as robust and resilient as it once was. Throughout this chapter you'll see data that reinforces that conclusion. It appears our over-all health as a nation has been in steady decline over the last four or five decades based on this country's relative life expectancy figures compared to other countries in the world since the mid-1980s. Timing wise, you can assume that through those decades, over 50 percent of our population could have lived through much of that change from age ten and up.

Focusing only on the most vulnerable populations that were identi-fied during this pandemic—the obese, diabetics, heart patients, and the immunocompromised—it was apparent that each of these conditions grew into serious threat levels since the 1960s, 1970s, and 1980s. There are no major solutions to these problems facing the American population on the horizon of which I'm aware, at least not right around the corner. So, risks from future pandemics become very real to the same popula-tions. Here are the conditions and the data showing the decline for each and when the decline intensified. Pay attention to the dates.

As the experts stated, one of those groups at the highest risk for COVID-19 deaths was the obese. Obesity became recognized in the 1970s with a sharp surge showing up in 1976, and it has not stopped ris-ing since then. (7)

Also at an identified risk were diabetics. The head of the CDC in 1994 declared that diabetes had reached epidemic promotions and in 2019 had become the fifth-leading cause of death in the US. (8)

Cardiovascular disease was one more condition identified as posing a risk, although conventional medicine's efforts have dramatically reduced death rates since the 1980s, when the condition peaked in the mid-1960s. Heart disease, however, remains the leading cause of death in the United States. (9) Even someone on drugs for this condition would still be identified and considered in the comorbidity profile for a coronavirus.

Although the elderly were also at risk, age is a fact of life, and the healthier one ages, the less vulnerable they would become.

Finally, the immunocompromised—those people with tumors, blood-related malignancies like leukemia, organ transplant patients, those taking immunosuppressants, those with advanced or untreated HIV, and those taking high-dose corticosteroids—that group has grown in recent decades and is estimated at 3 percent of the population, or slightly over ten million people. (10)

Since the immunocompromised are the most complicated group mentioned, many of those identified with this condition became so because of scientific medicine's efforts to cure disease. Except for tumors and malignancies, which go way back, the others do not. I'm not saying those advances were a bad thing—they were just a thing.

Organ transplants weren't aggressively happening until the 1980s, although the first few were done in the late '60s. Prescribing immunosuppressant drugs didn't begin until the early '60s but most aggressively since 1983. HIV was first identified in the early 1980s. Everything that causes the population to become immunocompromised, besides just being born with a weak system, came into play forty to sixty years ago. (11)

Cortisone was first isolated in 1950, but today systemic corticosteroids are used in every medical specialty from dermatology, respirology, endocrinology, gastroenterology, hematology, rheumatology/immunology, and ophthalmology as well as for other specific conditions not falling into those categories. It's used throughout medicine. (12)

Again, noticing the dates, all the growth of cases, the technological advances exacerbating some conditions and the spikes causing concern occurred within that roughly forty- to fifty-year window. I couldn't help but draw the conclusion that over those years, we appear to have become less healthy. This begs the question, does the life expectancy of our nation also reflect that fact? In a chapter upcoming, you will see that it does, and as a result, our standing within the global community in terms of the longevity of our citizens, in comparison, has dramatically declined since the mid-1980s.

Weren't there other pandemics that came before COVID-19?

Amazingly, America survived many viral epidemics and pandemics without all the fear and drama being played out by the politicians, the media, and the institutional medical community as with this one. Here is a list of the five greatest epidemic or pandemic threats we faced prior to this one and managed to live through them all without complete devastation. Every one of them was caused by a virus.

In our lifetimes we faced the Asian flu (1957–58)—and yes, flu is caused by one of four influenza viruses, two of which cause seasonal flu and pandemics, one is circulated only in the animal population, and the fourth is very mild and doesn't cause epidemics.

Next was the Hong Kong flu (1968–70), then HIV/AIDS (1980–present) originating in Africa, and HIV, another virus. There was also SARS (2002–03) from China's Yunnan Province, and finally, the swine flu pandemic (2009–10)—all before the COVID-19 pandemic appeared in 2020. (13)

Through any of those epidemics or pandemics prior to COVID-19, did we lock down the country? Did we throw everyone into a panic? No, there was another way of handling each one.

Back then, the important communication occurred in a way that made problem-solving efficient and kept the patient/doctor relationship intact. Back then, we listened to our primary physicians, and they were educated through the normal professional network that was in place. Not so today. With COVID-19, the orders came from the top of the professional network directly to the patient and the independent physician without the flexibility they had always been given to treat as they saw fit.

This time, Dr. Fauci was America's doctor, and everybody looked to him for answers on what they should do, what they should take, when to go to the hospital, frankly on every aspect of the coronavirus issue.

Everything! Yet, had people realized that Dr. Fauci's background might not have qualified him to be the absolute expert on anything except the science of immunology or virology, they might not have taken him so seriously.

After Fauci's medical residency in 1968, he was immediately drafted to work at NIAID, where in 1974 he became head of the physiology section and in 1980 became chief of NIAID's Laboratory of Immunoregulation. Four years later, he was appointed director of NIAID, a position he has held ever since. His entire career has not been broad and seemed to always be isolated to immunology and virology. (14) So, with that many years of a sharply honed focus, it seems his perspective was limited, but that didn't matter. Fauci was king and everyone seemed to obey.

Yet, everything Fauci looked at he did so through the lens of *can we vaccinate against it?* This old saying, "When you're a hammer—everything looks like a nail" might truly have applied to Dr. Anthony Fauci in this case.

Although Dr. Fauci had an impressive background in one field, the fact still exists that he had zero experience on the front line treating patients with various therapeutics as clinical physicians do. Those professionals were finding anecdotal proof that there were therapeutic answers with efficacy, but that wasn't good enough for the medical, institutional leadership. There had to be a vaccine. So, while we waited over eight months for the vaccine miracle to happen, 336,000 people in the US died. (15)

Of course, there are more questions that need answering.

I could go on with questions forever, but I won't. I'll just list just a few of the big ones, and you can judge on your own if they've been answered to your satisfaction or not. Leaving questions like this hanging only perpetuates uncertainty, confusion, and frankly fear about whom to trust and what might happen in the future. Here are the big questions, in my mind.

Where and how did the virus really originate—so we can stop this from happening again?

Why did no one predict any potential collateral damage that might result to our children, small businesses, and our economy, for example, with the radical lockdown and isolation mandates?

What happened to informed consent for the vaccines? Not having informed consent has long been the basis for many malpractice claims: when a doctor performs a treatment or procedure without informed consent of the patient and without the patient being made aware of the risks prior, they are vulnerable. (16)

Continuing from the same source, there exists a patient's bill of rights, which is active in many states and, in fact, was ratified by the Supreme Court and which rejects a clinician-centered and paternalistic approach to consent, replacing paternalism with patient autonomy. What happened to its viability?

Even a court of law, for the most part, cannot force an adult to have medical treatment or a medical procedure if they chose not to. So, why is it perfectly fine for employers, schools, the military, and airlines, among other companies, to require employees to get these shots?

Why was natural immunity totally ignored by a medical profession, especially Dr. Fauci—when in prior years all medical professionals voiced just the opposite to be true? Why now are vaccines deemed more powerful than natural immunity? On this one alone, it's hard not to question motive.

Why is there no formal tracking method for adverse effects from the vaccines being collected from physicians other than the VAERS (Vaccine Adverse Event Reporting System), set up by the CDC and reliant on patient submissions? Their "reports may include incomplete, inaccurate, coincidental and unverified information." (17) That is the go-to database?

Why were pharmaceutical companies protected from legal action for adverse reactions to their vaccines or boosters for COVID-19 and subsequent variants with complete immunity?

The point of this chapter is to illustrate how inconsistencies in messaging, lack of accountability in answering related questions, and lack of transparency in the data all contributed to countless more questions. When we don't know what to believe, we begin to ask ourselves if we know who to believe either.

Chapter 3

WHO TO BELIEVE?
THAT'S NOW THE QUESTION

By mid-2022, it was becoming evident that the experts were losing credibility. Besides all the speculation about the effectiveness of the rollout, what was promised didn't happen. Some are now beginning to realize that maybe science, or at least their science, isn't perfect.

I promised to name names, so here are the people responsible for this misinformation nightmare. First was Rochelle Walensky, MD, head of the CDC, Francis Collins, MD, PhD, head of the NIH, Anthony Fauci, MD, head of NIAID, and Deborah Birx, MD, who had been named US Global Coordinator of the White House Task Force in 2020. Other players included the FDA and even the AMA, and although their leadership was not visible, they both functioned in supporting roles.

Is it fair to point fingers now? I believe it is because these were the people who provided all the facts, made all the scientific pronouncements, and really called the shots. Politicians and the media believed what was reported to them and based subsequent policy on that knowledge. Well, let me back up a bit. The CDC at this point played the lead role setting policy, although as I mentioned before, since we don't know how the gears function within the administrative state of government, Dr. Fauci or others might have been involved behind the scenes with policy too. The directives, however, were publicly led by the CDC.

I've recognized the failings and limitations of the medical establishment for some time, which is why I've continually had better results and why this is now my second book on finding health and healing options elsewhere. Still, the coronavirus crisis was so confusing in the beginning, the public needed a trusted voice. Now, that same public has begun to form their own opinions, is trying to deal with the resulting disappointment and eroding trust, and has woken up to how many lives were ruined by leaders who, for whatever reason, wouldn't change course.

In case you think I've been too harsh with these four MDs in leadership, I haven't. They are all now admitting, in one way or another, that they may have really screwed this up. One bailed early when shenanigans were leaked between the US and Wuhan lab—another one directly said they may have gotten it wrong, still another admits to lying to us, and the third has hightailed it out of Dodge before eventual accountability sets in. Here is the detail.

First, there was Dr. Francis Collins who stepped down from his position at the NIH just two weeks following the leaked documents that showed just how the US funneled federal funds into the Wuhan Institute of Virology for its gain-of-function research on coronaviruses. (18) Collins had headed the NIH for twelve years and will return to the National Human Genome Research Institute.

Next came Dr. Rochelle Walensky, the current head of the CDC, who admitted in mid-August 2022 that her agency may have gotten it wrong on the handling of COVID-19. She appeared in a variety of network interviews over that week stating that to try to fix things in the future, the organization would be going through a complete overhaul. In bureaucratic speak, that means they will be tweaking a few things and firing no one. Walensky herself is not stepping down. You can find three such videos from *CBS Mornings*, *Forbes*, and *The Hill TV* on YouTube under "Rochelle Walensky Mistakes."

The third is Dr. Deborah Birx, the White House Coronavirus Response Coordinator who was responsible for leading the team overseen by Vice President Mike Pence during the Trump administration. Birx revealed in her recent book published in April 2022, with no remorse, that she lied to the American public about COVID statistics. She was directly responsible for setting much of the public policy. To quote her verbatim from the book, "Our Saturday and Sunday report-writing routine soon became: write, submit, revise, hide, resubmit." And another direct quote referring to Birx admitting she deceived Trump to push COVID measures: "I couldn't do anything that would reveal my true intention." (19) Her book also reveals that when she and Dr. Scott Atlas, a frontline clinical physician another adviser to President Trump, were together with the president in the Oval Office, Atlas shared a different point of view with the president when asked about a particular aspect of this policy. Birx was furious and told him what she thought of him contradicting her in front of the president after the meeting. (20)

According to Rep. Andy Biggs, AZ, "Dr. Deborah Birx admitted in her new book that she falsified COVID data in order to advocate for lockdowns and other draconian measures. She destroyed our country from within." Posted on Twitter, July 18, 2022.

Last but not least, regarding the revealing evidence of this leadership abandoning ship—not because the pandemic is over but because they have or don't want egg on their faces. On August 22, 2022, Dr. Anthony Fauci, according to all major news outlets, is set to leave as director of NIAID and as chief medical adviser to President Joe Biden in December 2022. Fauci has served more than fifty years in government, and although he is eighty-one years of age, I would have guessed that his resignation would have more likely occurred at the end of Biden's term (2025) since another pandemic and vaccine effort could be on the horizon. This exit seemed rushed to me.

It's my opinion that the real reason for Fauci's abrupt departure is not a new career path opening up at his age but more likely the fact that if Republicans take the House of Representatives in November 2022, Senator Rand Paul (also an MD) has said he would hold hearings asking Fauci very pointed questions about his involvement in gain-of-function research (the origination of the virus through US grants made available), his hiding of the real origins of the pandemic (the Wuhan cover-up), and likely a few other topics Dr. Fauci would not want to address. In other words, timing is everything.

Medical leadership shut out prominent dissenting voices.

If you question the validity of one source, how do you verify or dismiss that source if you never hear another side? In this case, the other side was completely discredited. Since those voices never appeared on mainstream media, the public had to search elsewhere for medical mavericks who existed out in the weeds. And they were out there with another side of the overall COVID-19 strategy, but most people wouldn't work that hard to track them down.

One group was the frontline clinical physicians who were treating patients from the beginning of the coronavirus outbreak with success and merely wanted to share their therapies. The second group was composed of highly credentialed physicians who came from outside of government and were as notable in their professional achievements as those calling the shots in Washington. They were also more relevant.

There is no room here to list all the physicians who comprise the second group with their credits, so, for the purpose of this section, I'll make general references and then sprinkle in a few names throughout the book. You can note who they are and look them up to read what they have to say, if you are interested. They're extraordinarily smart but became persona non grata very quickly.

In all cases, these medical doctors with their different points of view were labeled science-deniers and immediately discounted and ridiculed by the institutional bureaucrats, who happened to be doctors too, but who hadn't treated patients in decades—or maybe ever. The media also slandered these professionals while social media deplatformed many or simply canceled them all together. They were scorned by other physicians who for one reason or another were influenced by the institutions who govern them.

As you remember, the group who set all directives were the academic, institutional, or government-employed physicians—many who dealt with research and operated in a completely different reality. They were thinkers, studiers, theorizers, and researchers of disease. They were either paid by the government or funded, partially or wholly, by grants from corporations, including pharmaceutical companies, making this group more likely to political influence and direct industry from many sources including the pharmaceutical industry. As a group, and because of the power their agencies wielded, they were also more susceptible to financial incentives. This group held the dominant voice in any conversation about this pandemic. They had all the power.

The maverick physicians were cut from a different cloth. They owed loyalty to no one; they were free thinkers and weren't afraid to speak up. Since they weren't allowed a stage in the public forum back then, patients remained in the dark about options that might have helped them recover more quickly or recover at all.

Soon many of these doctors had their profiles on Google edited, their Wikipedia pages slanderously rewritten, their social media access banned, and reputations sullied in the media. You can always tell the pioneers by the arrows in their backs. These were doctors like Scott Atlas, MD; Marty Makary, MD; Peter McCullough, MD; Robert Malone, MD; and others like Sherry Tenpenny, DO; Jane Ruby, PhD; Simone Gold, MD, JD, FABEM; and Christiane Northrup, MD, as well as many more. You might not agree with their opinions, but they all have notable credential and are worth listening to before you make decisions about them. These eight had differing opinions on just about everything the government was insisting.

Yet there were still many clinical physicians who agreed with the medical leadership in Washington, at least publicly, including many family doctors. Yes, the clinical faction was split, and although both sides had credentials, not all were mavericks.

The group of clinicians who agreed with Fauci, Birx, and Walensky may not have had much of a choice. Some were just trapped in the system that, believe it or not, governs most physicians either through direct influence or peer pressure. For some, it's because of policies and procedures established by the hospitals in which they hold privileges. For others it's the governance indirectly by the insurance providers (including Medicare and Medicaid) who reimburse their patient care and to whom their therapies are accountable. Additionally, some are at the mercy of the corporate entities (often hospital systems) who own their practices or clinics. So, many such clinical physicians are intimidated or influenced against testing or trying different therapeutics to begin with. This includes the use of off-label options, which required courage from the doctor to try.

To prove my point about government intimidation, the California state legislature passed a bill on August 25, 2022, that would allow regulators to punish physicians for spreading misinformation or disinformation related to COVID-19. Punishment could include suspending or revoking a physician's California medical license. Misinformation is defined as "false information that is contradicted by contemporary scientific consensus contrary to the standard of care." (21) That would include any opinions about vaccinations or treatments that weren't mainstream in the conventional medical world, including alternative options on off-label therapeutic use. Governor Gavin Newsom signed this bill into law.

It's no wonder many physicians continue to timidly retreat.

With masking the silent debate continues.

At the risk of beating a dead horse, I'm still stunned at how many in conventional medicine remain obstinate about masking—even though there has been so much credible criticism surrounding the policy. Some are so defiant I'm afraid we'll need to buckle up for the next epidemic because the craziness may not be over.

Quite early in the pandemic, dozens of clinical physicians began speaking out against the efficacy of mask wearing for viruses and even certified industrial hygienist Stephen Petty testified on the subject ("Why Masks Don't or Can't Work" [April 1, 2020]), to the New Hampshire state senate citing extensive randomized controlled trials, studies, and meta-analysis reviews of these studies, all showing that masks and respirators do not work to prevent respirator influenza-like illnesses or respiratory illnesses believed to be transmitted by droplets and aerosol particles since especially in viral respiratory diseases, the aerosol particles are too fine to be blocked. (22) This was a lengthy explanation but a scientifically based point of view our leadership didn't want to hear at the time.

More and more articles appeared citing data from other countries, history with pandemics and the like resulting in the conclusion the *Wall Street Journal* drew in their opinion piece on August 18, 2022, which was titled: "Fauci and Walensky Double Down on Failed Covid Response—Lockdowns were oppressive and deadly. But US and WHO officials plan worse for the next pandemic." The article further stated, "For all the talk from officials like Dr. Fauci about following 'the science," these leaders ignored decades of research—as well as fresh data from the pandemic—when they set strict Covid regulations." (23)

Even with the overreach on this issue, the public realized the downside that was occurring. We were further separating people by masking their emotions, hiding their smiles, and hindering the development of young children who were just commencing their socialization and early verbalization skills. What we did to our children's development was unforgiveable to me.

Still, with the pronouncement last summer from Dr. Rochelle Walensky (CDC), who acknowledged with her blanket statement that maybe they got it wrong, there are still enough believers out there who will react even more irrationally when the next pandemic hits, evident by another article that appeared two years after the onset.

On April 11, 2022, an article appeared in todaysparent.com titled: "Should your child wear a mask at school? Most kids in Canada no longer need to wear masks at school, but many health experts say wearing one is still a good idea. Here's how to decide what's right for your family." The article in *Today's Parent* continues to outline why masks are great, effective, and encouraged. (24)

When such lingering debate continues, it's up to everyone to use their own common sense and not let fear control their decision-making on this issue or any other.

Who's right on off-label use?

One of the most violent debates among physicians was about whether therapeutics might be warranted or not to cure early coronavirus cases. There were clinical physicians initially advocating for hydroxychloroquine in combination with antibiotics and zinc as an effective therapeutic trio, and soon others joined the chorus of therapeutic options. Not long after, others began touting the effectiveness of Ivermectin—both off-label drugs that had been approved decades prior, were affordable, readily available, and basically safe for use. The medical leadership was immediate and harsh in their criticism of both.

While the leadership insisted that all these therapeutics were useless, unproven, or very dangerous to use, that same leadership would not provide any other consideration of a therapeutic option, and we were told we must wait for the miracle vaccines to become available at the end of the year. The therapeutic debate, by the way, occurred in March of 2020, early enough to have saved lives, but the leadership's edict was absolute, and it was based on "science."

While the public waited, unable to get prescriptions for therapeutics that might have saved lives, people died. By the time the first vaccine was released to the public on December 11, 2020, it was reported that the pandemic had already killed 290,000 in the US and nearly 1.6 million people worldwide. (25) The death statistic reported early was through the year-end 2020, so it is greater than this one. They are still horrific numbers, and although some frontline doctors tried to speak out about earlier options, their voices were silenced.

One example was a doctor in New York: Vladimir Zelenko, MD, was one of the first in the country to successfully treat thousands of COVID-19 patients in the prehospital settling with a cocktail that included hydroxychloroquine. He did so while battling recurrent and metastatic sarcoma, recovering from open-heart surgery, and undergoing aggressive chemotherapy. His now-famous "Zelenko Protocol" saved lives all around the world. He was ignored and discredited at the time. He has since died. (26)

Additionally, the moment President Trump mentioned hydroxychloroquine, because that is one of the drugs he was also given and continued to take as a prophylactic, everyone in the media and medical leadership reacted hysterically. The idea was dismissed as ludicrous since hydroxychloroquine was a drug normally used to prevent malaria. Yes, it was an off-label drug, but it seemed to be working. You remember Trump left the hospital within three days and said he never felt better.

Later down the road Ivermectin was introduced as a likely answer by Pierre Kory, MD, a former specialist at the University of Wisconsin, and Mark Marik, MD, the former chief of critical care at Eastern Virginia Medical School. Later, hundreds of more clinical physicians joined their ranks in extolling the virtues of Ivermectin, but like hydroxychloroquine, Ivermectin would demonstrate an off-label use of a drug. Subsequently both drugs were denied application in hospitals or to be prescribed to pharmacies for this virus.

The off-label uproar regarding Ivermectin stemmed from the fact that although originally designed as an antiparasitic drug used in grazing animals, it was approved for use in humans in 1987 to treat parasitic infections. It is currently affordable at thirty to forty dollars a dose and has been used safely since for all these decades. That one, too, was forbidden for use by any patient in the US. (27)

An inconvenient use of an off-label drug like hydroxychloroquine or Ivermectin simply didn't fit the plan, so regardless of anecdotal field data that was all over the place submitted by physicians on the front lines treating patents, both drugs had to be ignored at least, and refuted at best. This begs the next topic.

Why banning off-label use is bogus.

Although the primary weapon of attack against these drugs was the excuse that a drug can't be used for another purpose just because it currently exists. That's not true, but they said it anyway.

Off-label application has rarely ever been questioned from a patient's health care provider since it's always been in the purview of the physician to determine whether a drug is medically appropriate for their patient or not—as long as it is currently on the market. There have never been such authoritarian measures against off-label use with drugs—especially in an emergency like we faced with COVID-19. Instead, this time, such drugs were banned for use on this virus, and instead of giving physicians the flexibility they were always awarded before, these drugs' uses were centralized with the FDA. Now, each needed reapproval for the applied use, which the FDA had no intention of granting.

Examples of off-label drug use are everywhere in medicine since it's quite common for chemotherapy drugs to be used off-label for various forms of cancer if the physician thinks it's viable. Additionally, nobody in medicine turned up their noses when Viagra was switched for use as a miracle erectile dysfunction drug even though its original purpose was to lower blood pressure. Or when Rogaine, the hair restoration medicine, was found to be effective in hair growth even though it was originally intended as a blood pressure treatment. Nope, because sales increased for the pharmaceutical companies who owned the original patents to both.

Could there have been another reason for discounting off-label therapeutics?

There was very likely another reason for keeping therapeutics off the market—a financial imperative. The pharmaceutical companies who developed these vaccines had already invested billions and decades of research trying to perfect mRNA drugs for some application, and finally the pandemic appeared. They instantly focused on coronaviruses, so why in the world would these companies encourage any therapeutic that already existed at a cost of thirty dollars a dose to be used in place of the vaccine that could make them bundles?

Pharmaceutical companies are in the business of making money first, helping humanity second. Please note that I didn't say the people employed by these companies have the same motives, I said the companies themselves. Any company that's publicly traded must answer quarterly to their shareholders, and a worldwide pandemic of this magnitude presents a potential windfall to companies like Pfizer.

Besides, the American public has been conditioned to look to pharmaceutical companies for the answer to almost every health-related issue, the coronavirus event being no exception. So, passing on therapeutics for a new wonder vaccine would easily be accepted. If you think that's an exaggeration, the trajectory of Big Pharma's revenues demonstrates that point precisely. When we look at Big Pharma's revenues over the last twenty years (all companies), they increased more than 400 percent. The worldwide pharmaceutical market revenues in 2001 were $390.2 billion, but twenty years later in 2021, they grew to $1.424 trillion. (28) Yes, that is trillion with a *t*.

Pfizer alone, the leading COVID vaccine supplier, had total revenues in 2020 of $41.7 billion, and in 2021 that rose 95 percent to a whopping $81.3 billion. (29) That dramatic increase wasn't because of an uptick in Chantix or Premarin sales.

The other reason for withholding therapeutics.

The third rationale for therapeutics being ignored was to justify the need for a vaccine in the first place! If there were already therapeutics on the market that were safe, inexpensive, and working effectively against a threatening disease, there would be no need for the FDA to approve a vaccine for that same disease. Who would ever buy one or even want one?

At least that was the policy back in the good old days, when the polio vaccine and measles, mumps, and rubella (MMR) vaccines were developed. Back then, in all cases, there was no proven therapeutic on the market for any of those conditions and they all posed imminent risks to the public. Of course, vaccines made sense then.

Today, times have changed. The pharmaceutical industry is a multibillion-dollar industry with undeniable influence over the field of medicine. Here's a little history on why pharmaceutical companies may have wanted these mRNA vaccines on the market now.

The potential for mRNA vaccines had been a glimmer in the eye of scientists since 1970 and later the 1990s when the first mRNA flu vaccine was tested in mice. In humans, the first tests were in 2013, but that vaccine was for rabies. The delay was due to the degrading factor that occurred before spreading the spike protein into human cells. The testing, however, continued with so much of this groundwork being laid well before COVID-19 hit. (30)

Continuing from that article, the mRNA vaccine was still in laboratories for decades with pharmaceutical companies testing potential applications that included possible treatments for cancer too. It seems like the mRNA discovery was a potential product looking for a viable purpose. It was hanging out there with various pharmaceutical companies filing patents and trying applications when COVID-19 appeared! This epidemic provided the perfect test market for proving the efficacy of a drug application that was never approved for use in humans until August 12, 2021, long after it was introduced for public use in December 2020. (30)

Tests could now be run on massive amounts of people, and they'd have the data they needed to refine the product, adapt it for future variants of COVID-19, and who knows what else? But would the results ever be revealed to the public or published in medical journals? We all know the answer to that question.

So, while we're deciding who to believe, in hindsight, I think we need to include Big Pharma in the mix of individuals directing the game plan since they were clearly leaning on everyone. Therefore, do I believe anything the pharmaceutical industry tells me today? I absolutely do not.

Why would some argue against the benefit of supplements?

Professionals can choose sides by one side withholding data. Again, the two primary camps surface—institutional medicine and other physicians treating patients. The benefits of supplementing the immune system with certain vitamins and minerals has been known for decades but not exposed to the public unless people dug for it, until recently with the COVID-19 experience. Even then, the information to the public originated from the bottom up, not the top down. We heard the news first from physicians on the front line, who know patients best and hopefully people were able to figure out that adding those supplements was affordable and easy to do.

There was one study that revealed that 80 percent of COVID-19 patients were vitamin D deficient (31). With reports like this, people were now understanding that folks with weaker immune systems might be more likely to contract the virus.

Unable to ignore the data surrounding vitamin D deficiency, the scientific medical community finally got on board, and a few of them mentioned this vitamin to us in media interviews. That was nice to see even though their history has been to totally ignore supplementation in the public arena.

The reasons people are deficient in vitamin D vary—for some, it's living in parts of the country that receive less sunshine, and for others, the color of their skin plays a role—those with high melanin (darker skin) are less able to receive the sun's healthy rays. Even if people do reside in sunbelt states and have limited exposure to direct sunlight, deficiency can still be an issue based on their amount of exposure. Poor diet can also contribute to the statistic.

Deficiencies range from 70 to 80 percent in some groups. Some studies state that vitamin D deficiency is as great as 80 percent within the US population with the worldwide average deficit being closer to 75 percent.

With all the information that exists and the fact that our immune systems are critical to our health, you'd think the experts would have acknowledged the value of this extraordinary function of the human body. But conventional, scientific medicine is so focused on external fixes they ignore the most basic elements of healthy living: prevention and what the patient can do to keep themselves well.

The scientific medical community ignored the need for zinc too. Even though the first sentence in the abstract of an article titled "Zinc deficiency and immune function" from the *National Library of Medicine* states, "Zinc deficiency can have marked effects on virtually all components of the immune system." (32) Still, physicians couldn't be bothered translating that information into strong immune system reminders that even could be posted on CDC.gov or other websites to keep people healthy.

So, if they're not completely ignoring us, they are refusing to acknowledge that people can really help themselves without running to the doctor with disease after disease and requiring drug after drug. Here is an example of naysayers who held their ground. In February 2021, the Cleveland Clinic newsroom published an article that said, and I quote, "Recent research shows popular immune health supplements, vitamin C and zinc are no match for COVID-19." (33) They also included vitamin C in their statement, which is equally ridiculous since this vitamin also has proven immune-strengthening benefits, but there's no room here to quote the many such studies.

There are two reasons why their testing might not confirm the efficacy of supplementation. The first is that these institutions don't understand routine dosages from therapeutic dosages. If a person is deficient or their immune system is struggling, the therapeutic dosage is required. So, a person who is truly deficient in a vitamin or mineral needs to take more than the minimum daily requirement. Researchers should be aware of that in their testing too. Obviously, they aren't. Or maybe they didn't want supplements to work so they plugged in moderate doses. I don't doubt a thing when it comes to attempts to discredit natural methods for healing—that's been going on for decades.

Anyway, ask any holistic MD, osteopath (DO), licensed naturopath, or chiropractor, and a variety of other more naturally focused providers, and they can explain maintenance doses versus therapeutic doses to you. I'm healthier than I've ever been after forty years of off-and-on health challenges. I don't take anywhere near the recommended daily requirement.

The second reason why some of the prestigious medical journals as well as organizations like the AMA still flatly deny the benefit of supplements—saying there is no proof that vitamin C, vitamin D3, zinc, or any other supplement is effective against disease. That shows their ignorance and lack of understanding of what these supplements are supposed to be doing.

As I've stated before, supplements aren't designed to kill the diseases, as their drugs are, instead supplements are designed to supplement the body's immune system and help strengthen it so the immune system can do the killing. Physicians are conditioned to using external products to do the work, like drugs. They don't understand how to simply help the body do the job it was designed to do so the work gets done through internal mechanisms.

So how do people ever know who to believe?

The first test I use for deciding who to believe and who not to is how much they care about you versus how much they care about themselves. That has to do with their posturing, including how truthful they are about their limitations and how often they try to bluff. A person's health is too serious an issue for bluffing, discrediting others, or insisting they're right. Any of those behaviors indicate to me their lack of confidence or a hidden agenda, and in either case, it's about them.

Another red flag for me is if they're defensive, if they make excuses, or if they blame other people. Again, that's when their stock goes down in my book. Also, if they try to intimidate and bully instead of persuade, I disconnect. In medicine, there should be logical arguments presented and the patient's concerns respected.

Finally, people who continually repeat something to make themselves more impressive or believable always remind me of quote from Shakespeare's *Hamlet*, Act III, Scene ii. "Thou dost protest too much, methinks." In the case of the "based on science" line we heard over and over, they weren't protesting too much, but they sure were insisting too much that you don't question anything they say. To me that was two sides of the same coin.

With all that said, I never put my total trust in another person, regardless of how educated the person might be. I might trust that person to give me advice, educate me about pros and cons of an issue or subject. I might seek out more than one knowledgeable resource and even read a little about the subject myself. When push comes to shove, however, after I've asked plenty of questions and looked at all sides of the issue—I always make the final decision myself, and I own that decision.

Just remember, when it comes to MDs, some are by-the-book conventional medical, pharmaceutically focused and in need of scientific proof for everything. Others consider anecdotal evidence worth considering too. These doctors are a little more creative and are out-of-the-box thinkers. I happen to prefer the latter group who tend to be more enlightened and open to new ideas. I tend to listen to them more frequently before I finally decide.

Chapter 4

YOU CAN ALWAYS BELIEVE RESULTS

I've always been results oriented. When I started my advertising agency back in the early 1970s, as the first woman in Arizona to do so, I obviously had very little credibility. Forget being the first of something, just being a woman entrepreneur in those days created doubts. I had to work twice as hard to be taken seriously. Long story short, my little firm ended up delivering remarkable results for clients, and that's how we grew. We doubled in size seven times during the first fourteen years, so people noticed. The results my firm achieved for clients drew attention too. That's also how I learned how important results were.

Results became how my firm grew and was how I marketed my firm to potential clients. In presentations I'd show the dramatic results we had achieved for other clients and how little we spent. That, by the way, was unusual in the advertising business in those days. Most agencies sold their creativity and the clever campaigns they implemented for their clients. I was just different and led with strategy—the creative came later. That's why we were so successful, even for a small company.

Eventually, I was asked to bring the same strategically focused, results-oriented methodology I used to generate magic for clients of my advertising agency to corporations both nationally and internationally. No question, results mattered then, and they do today.

So, imagine my shock when I heard my rheumatologist tell me my newly acquired rheumatoid arthritis was a chronic condition. Chronic, you realize, means that a condition will continue for a long duration, perhaps forever, and if it does subside, it is due to reoccur. To show how normal this is in medicine, according to NIH, "Chronic diseases are among the most prevalent and costly health conditions in the United States. Nearly half (approximately 45 percent or 133 million) of all Americans suffer from at least one chronic disease." (34)

That word was hard for me to accept since I was a problem solver by nature. Chronic? *Impossible*, I thought, *there's an answer for everything*. And of course there was since I managed to recover from rheumatoid arthritis, leukemia (twice), chronic allergies, hyperthyroidism, psoriasis, and neutropenia all outside of a profession that didn't always look for answers but instead was comfortable with chronic labels and treating symptoms. From then on, I was careful how much I trusted the scientific medical community and listened intently but never automatically followed all their advice or believed everything I was told. The diagnosis, yes, but past that everything else was up for grabs.

I do give a lot of credit to the extraordinary parts of conventional medicine that exist, for example their diagnostic capability, orthopedic surgical excellence, and transplant breakthroughs. I admire all the surgical mastery and a few other specialties in which they excel. But for routine care, especially for chronic conditions, there were too many drugs for me. Even some drugs caused additional symptoms, which required even more drugs.

Over the years, I always thought comprehensively to solve problems. With advertising campaigns there was always a mix of vehicles and methods to reach the consumer because their lifestyles were all over the place, so we had to be just as flexible and strategic with our messaging. I approached my health the same way. The body is so complex and integrated that isolating my healing program to only one approach seemed shallow and ineffective. I guess that's why mind-body-spirit medicine resonated with me. It works like the body works with what we think and believe determining the behavior that affects our physical selves, as well as how our emotions can directly weaken our immunity. Anyway, it's all too complex for the quick fix of a pill. I'm obviously right because pills continue to be sold and chronic illness keeps growing.

So, throughout my life, I looked for people like me, who were focused on eventual results.

It's easy to tell who delivers real results and who doesn't.

The recent pandemic showed the true colors many of the leaders anointed within the federal bureaucracy to lead us—be it politically or scientifically. In this case, we were routinely told the wrong thing—perhaps out of ignorance or because there was another agenda.

After Joe Biden was elected president, he promised the vaccine would end COVID-19 if enough people were vaccinated. Dr. Anthony Fauci, too, promised the vaccine would be the eventual solution to the spread of this coronavirus. Everyone promised that over and over, yet it didn't happen because we saw case after case of vaxxed people contracting COVID-19. That was not a case of positive results.

Only later did we discover that the vaccine really wasn't expected to prevent the virus (as most are) but only to mitigate symptoms and lessen the impact. Not the original promise. That was dishonest from the beginning and could have encouraged therapeutics and saved lives if they had been more transparent initially.

This was particularly upsetting to me when Anthony Fauci said as late as May 2021 when appearing on CBS's *Face the Nation*, when he was asked what would happen once a person received the vaccine, he still insisted the vaccine would stop the spread:

"In other words, you become a dead end to the virus. And when there are a lot of dead ends around, the virus is not going to go anywhere." (35)

Fauci was promising that vaccinating a good portion of the population would simply kill the spread of COVID-19. That was all based on science, once again. His comment was absolute, meaning once a person gets the vaccine, that is where the contagion stops, so they can't affect others and they will remain safe themselves.

Credibility finally flew out the window when, well into 2022, after taking the maximum doses of the vaccine and all the boosters, both Biden and Fauci contracted COVID-19 themselves. In fact, even after President Biden was given Paxlovid, Pfizer's new therapeutic to cure the coronavirus, he remained infected and continued to test positive, until after four tests covering multiple days, he finally tested negative. So much for results.

Still people continued to worship Dr. Fauci, and the media hung on every word. I was always skeptical. And now that "science" has retired, it's time to broaden our perspective past one man's opinion to include those from other medical scholars and practicing physicians with no ulterior motives, hidden agendas, or obvious egos.

Now it's time to absorb all the information that exists from many different sources and form our own conclusions. Results should still be the standard, and even though perfection isn't expected, public reporting and accountability toward some stated goal should be.

Old-fashioned vaccines and their results.

The old-fashioned vaccines from decades ago seemed to work better. We all remember when we received our polio vaccines as kids. We never got polio. Then, we were also given the MMR vaccine, and guess what again? We didn't get measles, mumps or rubella either. We also received diphtheria, tetanus, and whooping cough shots. Again, nobody seemed to contract those diseases as kids—or even later.

Overall, these old-style vaccines were amazingly effective over the long term, not requiring reinjection every few months. The polio vaccine, for example, which prevented the illness 90 percent of the time with the first two doses and 99 percent to 100 percent after the final third according to CDC data, worked. In terms of the MMR vaccine, again the CDC states that one dose is 93 percent effective, two doses of this vaccine result in 97 percent effectiveness against measles (37) and 88 percent effectiveness against mumps. (37) Again, impressive. It's different today.

How are today's vaccines working?

I think Dr. Deborah Birx sums it up nicely regarding the efficacy of the COVID-19 vaccines. In a direct quote from an interview she gave on video on July 24, 2022: "I knew these vaccines were not going to protect against infection," she continued, "And I think we overplayed the vaccines, and it made people then worry that it's not going to protect against severe disease and hospitalization. It will. But let's be very clear: 50 percent of the people who died from the omicron surge were older, vaccinated." (38) Completely contrary to what they were claiming well into the start of that year while they were pushing vaccines on every American with a pulse.

Of course, like everything else, when the pharmaceutical companies start heading in one direction, they rarely slow down. Now that more data is being revealed and the vaccine's effective life is limited and as the virus mutates, boosters are now being given—not one, not two, not three, but a total of four as of the writing of this book in September of 2022. These can be administered within two months of each other. There's nothing I can say since it's difficult to comment with a total jaw drop.

So, results be damned. If something isn't working too well, just keep trying and trying until you get it right—regardless of side effects inflicted on the testing population, which nobody can deny are happening.

Are poor results due to how the mRNA vaccines work?

First, these new vaccines shouldn't be labeled vaccines in the first place because they are constructed differently. I'm not sure what they are—you can judge for yourself.

> With mRNA vaccines, instead of injecting a weakened version of the virus, the vaccine introduces a package of genetic material called messenger RNA. This can be best understood as a set of instructions for producing some specific characteristic of the targeted (in the case of this vaccination, it's SARS-CoV-2's distinctive spike protein). This mRNA enters a few cells in the body and causes them to produce protein encoded in the instructions. The immune system then attacks this protein, learning the profile of the SARS-CoV-2 in the process. (39)

In other words, it's much like writing a program for a computer. The immune system attacks the foreign invader (the spike protein), and in doing so, it learns the profile of SARS-CoV-2 in the process. This process is completely synthetic and is an effort of science to replicate the normal function of the natural immune response to this foreign invader. In other words, they've inserted a middleman. Since the targeting (or programming) is to a particular strain, the vaccine focuses the immune system where it wants it to address but in the process has the likelihood to compromise the individual's immunity in other areas it might normally or simultaneously function.

So, explaining the mRNA shots further, it appears that when another strain of COVID appears later, there is no recognition and no natural immune response—making the patient more likely to contract that specific variation. It also necessitates individuals receiving yet another vaccine to address that new variant. Since those boosters now can be administered as closely as two months after the other, it all seems too erratic to me and demonstrates how the pharmaceutical companies are still gathering data on how these mRNA shots are behaving, and with no prior testing on humans or potential side effects, it's somewhat of a crapshoot.

I encourage readers to do their own research. I have a few suggestions below.

Other sources for researching the results of these vaccines and alternative therapeutics.

There are excellent physicians who bring differing opinions and more detail about the vaccines, their function, and their efficacy, as well as which therapeutics work including recent testing on all those issues that has occurred here and around the world. Sadly, there is little reported in the United States since the drug companies themselves have not been transparent about the detailed ingredients, testing, or reporting results. Other medical professionals do have access to some forms or research data.

There is Dr. Marty Makary, professor at Johns Hopkins University School of Medicine, best-selling author, and public health expert who hosts a podcast titled *A Second Opinion with Marty Makary*. Frankly, I'm not sure of his exact positions, but I know he is guest on Fox News occasionally. He has excellent credentials and seems measured in his responses.

Dr. Peter McCullough is a cardiologist and the former vice chief of internal medicine at Baylor University Medical Center. McCullough is the editor in chief and senior executive editor of two distinguished journals of cardiology, and his own work has exceeded over one thousand publications. McCullough hosts an Apple podcast titled *The McCullough Report*. He has been raked over the coals by the medical establishment and is a firm supporter of several therapeutics. He is very controlled in his responses as well. In fact, most of these physicians do not seem "on the fringe."

Scott Atlas, MD, a senior fellow in health care policy at the Hoover Institution of Stanford University, is another good source, and although he operates outside of the federal government bureaucracy, he was a special adviser to the president and a member of the White House Coronavirus Task Force led by Deborah Birx, MD. The two of them clashed. You can find Atlas on many YouTube videos, for example.

Women will absolutely appreciate the perspective of Christian Northrup, MD. Dr. Northrup has been a preeminent expert on women's health as an OBGYN in New England for many decades, is a *New York Times* best-selling author, and hosts *True North* on Substack. She happened to endorse my first *Get Well* book. She's one of the medical mavericks, is brilliant, and talks about issues for women nobody else does like the danger the mRNA vaccines pose to young women's reproduction. Dr. Northrup is a little more impassioned in her remarks, but her knowledge is unquestionable, and her data is solid. All these physicians appear regularly on other well-known podcast shows, some on cable television, and you can visit their individual websites too.

Dr. Northrup and the physicians who follow are all more controversial than the first three since this group has accessed countless more research on side effects and risks associated with these shots. If you want even more details, Northrup and the following physicians are the ones to investigate.

Dr. Robert Malone, a vaccine scientist who in the late 1980s was instrumental in establishing the original mRNA vaccine technology used in the Pfizer-BioNTech and Moderna COVID-19 vaccines. He also writes on *Who Is Robert Malone*, which appears on Substack. He is controversial because of his appearance on Joe Rogan's show when he quoted Professor Mattias Desmet of Ghent University in Belgium on mass formation psychosis. The mass formation theory created an uproar, although both

Desmet and Malone are more than well credentialed, and their information is rock solid. Even though Dr. Malone was vaccinated, he is clearly an advocate now about the risks associated with these vaccines.

There is also Simone Gold, MD, JD, FABEM, founder of America's Frontline Doctors, who has recently formed a telemedical nonprofit called GoldCare.com, which is designed to restore the patient-physician relationship and patient choice, breaking the paradigm of government and insurance control over individuals' health care decisions. I have never used them, but they are worth exploring.

The last two: Sherri Tenpenny, DO, is a neuromusculoskeletal medicine specialist in Cleveland, OH with over thirty-eight years in the medical field. She went viral after her testimony at a COVID-19 vaccine hearing. She opposes vaccination and the established scientific consensus. And Jane Ruby, PhD, host of *The Dr. Jane Ruby Show*, is a medical professional and a pharmaceutical drug development expert with over twenty years' experience in regulatory processes for drug approval with the FDA. With two doctoral degrees and a master's degree in nursing and international health economics, she is also a lightning rod on the issue regarding this virus, the subsequent vaccines, and their short-term and long-term negative effects.

They are all interesting and worth listening to in order to gain perspective on what the other side thinks.

The results are still being evaluated on all the domestically used vaccines (mRNA, viral vector type—such as Johnson & Johnson) and whether any cause serious side effects or even death. My point being still nobody knows the long-term effects since they've only been administered since December 2020 and more information is uncovered weekly—even though most of the data is withheld from the public or at least not being reported quickly and accurately.

What about the results hospitals achieved treating coronavirus patients?

Let's begin with the results that occurred since the pandemic first hit in spring of 2020. At this point the CDC was driving medical protocols for

US hospitals in COVID-19 cases because of the declared emergency. Still, patients continued to die while receiving the hospital care most assumed would save them.

Although many patients experienced sore throat, headache, diarrhea, nausea or vomiting, loss of small or taste, they were encouraged to wait until a fever above 100.4, a new cough, or new shortness of breath occurred. They were not encouraged to seek urgent care or hospital care until their symptoms were more severe, including having trouble breathing, experiencing pain or pressure in the chest, bluish lips, or feeling confused. (40)

There was no home testing available or widespread testing at the time due to a shortness of kits, among other reasons. Other reasons for delays in seeking doctor referrals to a hospital involved the inability to test prior to the doctor visits and the fact that tests from one's physician were taking three to five days at a time to deliver results. So, many days and perhaps weeks passed. During that time, patients had no treatment protocols at their disposal except for fluids and rest in a home environment. Personal physicians were not dispensing any type of therapeutic for the most part, so all of these factors caused delays before patients ended up in hospitals.

Once they were admitted, there were other factors at play. Ventilator use in hospitals was also questioned early, but hospitals continued to use them. According to an article in WebMD, on April 15, 2020, "But, the ventilator also marks a crisis point in a patient's COVID-19 course, and questions are now being raised as to whether the machines can cause harm too." The article went on to say: "Experts estimate that between 40% and 50% of patients die after going on ventilation, regardless of the underlying illness. It's too early to say if this is higher with COVID-19 patients, although some regions like New York report as many as 80% of people infected with the virus die after being placed on ventilation." (41)

Other early data was also alarming. Although a study regarding a hospital system in New York was published on WebMD early enough in this pandemic for physicians and hospitals to be able to adjust their strategy after reviewing it, I don't believe dramatic changes were made. The report was dated April 2020 and said: "The study included health records of 5,700 COVID-19 patients hospitalized between March 1 and April 4 at facilities overseen by Northwell Health, New York State's largest health system. Among the 2,634 patients for whom outcomes were known, the overall death rate was 21%, but it rose to 88% for those who received mechanical ventilation, the Northwell Health COVID-19 Research Consortium reported." (42)

Now, in all fairness, it could be because those patients were more serious, but dozens of highly experienced clinical physicians cited that the effects of COVID-19 on the human lung present more like altitude sickness than pneumonia, and the ventilators, in such a case, prove counterproductive. Although scientific medical institutions dismiss that claim on the grounds that altitude sickness drugs would be dangerous for COVID-19 patients, that's a false equivalence since no frontline physician group was advocating for the use of altitude sickness drugs, only increased oxygen therapy.

There was still enough controversy, even from family physicians, about how early ventilation therapy should start and if it should be used at all. Trying to sort all the data to be sure is above most people's paygrade; still, the debate over the first year on the issue of ventilation led many patients to question that therapy for themselves or loved ones.

Reimbursement may have skewed hospital protocols. See what you think.

This is an interesting point, so I did a little research and found an article regarding the reimbursement from Medicare that was also fact-checked. I am quoting from the Fact Check site. The article was titled "Hospitals get paid more if patients listed as COVID-19, on ventilators." This article appeared in *USA Today*. It continued, "Because if it's a straightforward, garden-variety pneumonia that a person is admitted to the hospital for— if they're Medicare—typically, the diagnosis-related group lump sum payment would be $5,000. But if it's COVID-19 pneumonia, then it's $13,000 and if that COVID-19 pneumonia patient ends up on a ventilator, it goes up to $39,000." (43)

How well did other hospital-based treatments work?

Ventilators weren't the only treatment protocol questioned for its efficacy either. Remdesivir is also controversial even though it is the only drug approved by the NIH and the FDA for COVID-19 as of the fall of 2022. That drug is the only one listed in the guidelines to hospitals published at covid19treatmentguidelines.nih.gov. However, remdesivir is not proven safe or effective.

Even the WHO recommended against remdesivir for hospitalized patients, regardless of disease severity, since there was no evidence that remdesivir improves survival or other outcomes. (44)

When the results are sketchy or contradictory, I always pause before blindly accepting what I'm being told—especially when it has to do with a drug with serious side effects or treatment protocols that could prove dangerous. One thing is certain, all these early treatment protocols, and even some adhered to today, demonstrate the *practice* of medicine in action—so anyone who believes scientific medicine is always perfect and harmless is dead wrong.

Why am I so critical?

I'm sure my tendency to question what I hear comes from a long history of realizing not every professional is correct in their assumptions 100 percent of the time, so I'd better make up my own mind. Even if they profess to be experts in a field, I believe them tangentially but not absolutely.

Of course, even our own viewpoints may be built on biases we don't even recognize. Some of those views are caused by limited exposure, a lack of curiosity, and even old beliefs we've never been able to shake. The next chapter will help us review some of those old beliefs or medical myths that have existed for decades. They may be right, or they may be wrong. That's up to you to decide.

Chapter 5
SHATTERING OLD MYTHS

Here's a question to ponder—is it possible that old beliefs you've held for years have kept you from getting well or staying well? I know that's a frightening concept, but it is possible for a person to be so blinded by strong beliefs that they have no ability to recognize even better opportunities that might present themselves.

When we were children, our parents were likely the major influence in the beliefs we formed, although peers and teachers also helped shape the foundation of what many of us still hold true today. Such ingrained beliefs have a lasting impact and contribute to our attitudes about people and key situations, but even more importantly, they help influence our behavior as well as what we attract into our lives.

Yes, it's possible for someone's belief system to contribute to all sorts of issues in their life—both good and bad. Think back about values you were taught as a kid, some based on slogans that made them easier to remember like: "Money is the root of all evil." "Blood is thicker than water." "It's who you know." And, of course, "Keep your nose to the grindstone." These and other teachings, often referred to as myths, often determine our eventual affluence and poverty, success and failure, and being happy or being a malcontent.

Your belief system can also determine whether you accept and live with a medical condition forever—because you were told you have to—or experience better health.

Our medical system is the best in the world.

This first myth is a powerful one that's been promulgated throughout society since World War II. We've all been told that the United States has developed the most magnificent system of medical care in the world, and since most of us believe that to be true, we continue to hold our doctors and the system that supports them in enormously high esteem. We believe our form of medicine is superior and ranks well above anything else—anywhere. Yet when we take a closer look at the facts, we find the truth is something totally different.

Let's take life expectancy, for example. Earlier, I brought up the possibility that we, in the United States, have become less healthy over the years. The data comparing the United States to the rest of the world through the end of 2019, or at the start of 2020, in our respective longevity confirms that. More recent data is now also showing that longevity in the United States has continued to decline even more so in the last two years, again more rapidly than the rest of the world, which I'll explain in the last chapter. Right now, the only detailed worldwide comparisons that are easy to understand exist in the study I'm quoting below. So, let's refer to that one initially.

The current life expectancy from birth and measured in years for both sexes for people living in the United States is 79.11 years. As good as that might look, it is not the envy of everyone else in the world. In fact, even though the number may seem high, comparatively it's not when you consider we rank close to Estonia and Cuba, both of whose populations live slightly longer, 79.18 years. Tragically, the United States ranks forty-sixth in longevity when compared to 194 other countries in the world. (45)

Continuing the analysis from that same data source, we fall short of forty-five other countries, including Hong Kong (85.29 years), which ranks number one; Japan (85.03 years) at number two; Italy (84.01 years) occupying the sixth position; Spain (83.99 years) at seventh; Australia (83.94 years) at eighth; France (83.13 years) at fourteenth; Canada (82.96 years); and Germany (81.88 years) at twenty-seventh. The United Kingdom (81.77 years) comes in at twenty-ninth. The real disheartening measure is when we realize countries we never hear about in terms of medical research or development like Mayotte, Maldives, French Guiana, Guam, Cyprus, Réunion, Slovenia, Guadeloupe, and Malta also have populations who live longer than we do.

This is even more shocking when we review data from eighteen years ago that appeared in the *Washington Post* in 2007: "A baby born in the United States in 2004 will live an average of 77.9 years. That life expectancy ranks 42nd, down from 11th two decades earlier, according to international numbers provided by the Census Bureau and domestic numbers from the National Center for health Statistics." (46)

Yes, you read that correctly. In 1984 we ranked eleventh in the world in terms of longevity, and then by 2004 we had fallen to forty-second (over a mere twenty-year period). Today, we're still dropping, and now, eighteen years later, we're down to forty-sixth. So, although our life expectancy chronologically has increased over time—from 77.9 in 2004 to 79.11—today, our overall health status in the world has continued to decline.

I want you to notice that this serious dip in our world standing began in the 1980s, which was forty-years ago, and we continue to head in the wrong direction! What does it matter how long we live if people in so many other countries live as many as 6.18 years longer on average than we do? This begs many questions, the most obvious being, why are we ranked so low?

There are several popular arguments offered by those in the medical field, and I will offer a counterpoint to each one of them, one at a time. The first being that it's the result of having a percentage of our population not covered by health insurance. As compelling an argument as that might sound, most individuals who are not covered by insurance still seem to get treatment—even for routine care at hospital emergency rooms where they're treated as charity cases and are never turned away. So, just because some people do not have health insurance does not mean they do not receive health care services.

The medical establishment also cites the obesity problem in the United States, which I'm sure most would blame on the fast-food restaurants on every corner. If people are ignorant about what good health care choices are, they make poor decisions. The stronger point being there is no preventive health care education available. We certainly can't point to poor socioeconomic conditions as a primary cause, which medical experts also cite, when we look at so many countries, not as affluent as the United States, ranking well above us in life expectancy.

The obvious excuse-makers also point to smoking, which is a silly argument given that "at least 40% of the population smokes, if not more… in South-East Asia, the Pacific islands and Europe—specially the Balkan region and also France Germany and Austria" (47) Most of those areas outrank us in life expectancy.

Medical experts also list homicides, opioid overdoses, and suicides, which may be valid but are collectively not enough to tip the scales as drastically as they are. Then they cite road accidents—really? Looking that up on Wikipedia's list of countries having the *most* traffic-related deaths, the US ranks 134th out of 182 countries. (48) That's low, not high.

There are two other considerations that aren't ever mentioned by our institutional medical community, but I'm sure you'll agree they contribute. The first is the fact that as a population, we overmedicate. We simply take too many pharmaceutical drugs—all of which produce one kind of side effect or another, and those effects often require more drugs. To confirm the fact, "between four and five billion prescriptions are filled each year in the United States." (49) Yes, billion. That's startling when we consider we only have a population of 338,343,549 people.

Although we can't statistically conclude that taking massive amounts of pharmaceutical drugs lowers our longevity rate, it seems likely.

The second point that I believe justifies our poor outcomes in how long we live, comparably, is that people in other countries are more accepting of and have more access to alternative forms of health care. For that reason, those individuals likely make better personal choices in the care they select and when.

A quick glance back at the countries that surpass us in years don't overmedicate with pharmaceuticals (as we appear to), they may not give in to radical treatments as quickly, and they may focus on prevention more. Patients in those countries appear to be more "alternative medicine" friendly, as you'll see in a minute, and practice a healthier lifestyle such as walking, eating fresh foods, and so on. To reinforce my point, if you've traveled much around the world or read anything about alternative care and its roots, you'll realize that alternative modalities are more prevalent in the United Kingdom, Europe, and Asia because their governments don't discourage their populations from looking beyond allopathic (conventional medical) methods for treatment as I illustrate below.

When traveling to any European country such as France and Germany, exterior signs on pharmacies that say "allopathic" on one side and "homeopathic" on the other are everywhere. Inside you'll find all kinds of homeopathic and herbal remedies. In Great Britain some pharmacies are allopathic and others, called medicinaries, are homeopathic. In fact, the royal family has used homeopathy for generations. If you don't believe me, google it.

In the US, a person has to visit a health food store or natural grocery store, which lacks a little in credibility for health care answers, to find alternative remedies including only a tiny portion of one shelf dedicated to homeopathic remedies. To find an expanded assortment of homeopathic remedies, one must visit a homeopathic provider to access their private medicinary, which is generally on-site. Unfortunately, homeopathic doctors aren't available everywhere.

Conventional medicine is much safer than any other method of care.

Here's another myth that could stand a little review. We all assume our allopathic system of medicine will protect us and keep us well and certainly not kill us, right? But just because we've held this belief for ages doesn't mean it's accurate.

I relied on the old quote "First, do no harm" to reinforce my belief in early years that my conventional medical physician's care was my insurance of safe treatment. The phrase is said to have originated from the ancient Greek Hippocratic oath, but no translations of that oath contain the specific language. Still, Hippocrates, the Father of Medicine from the fifth century BCE, used language very similar suggesting that the physician should not cause physical or overall harm to a patient. That was close enough for me.

If we want to be technically correct, the first published version of "do no harm" originated in medical texts from the mid-nineteenth century, so the seventeenth century English physician Thomas Sydenham gets credit for that. Regardless of who said what, I always thought somewhere in medical school that age-old philosophy was the core of what our medical doctors believed. I'm not sure that's the case anymore. I don't believe physicians have ever intentionally set out to harm their patients, but their mission got misaligned along the way. It's now more focused on saving lives, regardless.

History confirms this fact since today's field of medicine has dramatically changed from the days when the faithful family physician got to know us personally and understood what else might have been a contributor to our illness. They pretty much treated the whole person. Instead, this is now an era of specialization where physicians treat one body part or another. They focus on dermatology, osteopathy, pulmonology, gastroenterology, surgery, urology, and so on. The pay is better performing specialty care, and I suppose status is somewhat elevated as a result.

Still, when the trend in generalized medicine began to disappear, the American physician died right along with it, and what we have now is segmented care, less concerned about the whole patient than before. The greater perspective comes from the institutionalized viewpoint where edicts come from on high, treatment protocols are determined by the reimbursement from insurance companies or the federal government through Medicare and Medicaid, and hospitals continue to gobble up private practices thereby furthering collective standardization in a system that was always more personalized and individualized in their methodology. Every organization's priority must be met, so the patient doesn't come first any longer.

The shift away from patient-centered care has been gradually replaced by a war against the disease. In a quest to conquer the enemy and win at all costs, we now hear the medical professions referring to "killing" the germs, "fighting" the bacteria, "attacking" the virus, "wiping out" the cancer, and similar terminology, which clearly describes where the focus of conventional medicine now lies. They are at war with the invaders, and in each ongoing battle the collateral damage done to the patient's body becomes secondary to winning the war itself.

This seek-and-destroy mission encourages many if not most doctors to jump to radical, invasive treatments right off the bat and prescribe highly toxic and damaging drugs to treat even minor ailments. In an environment like that, and because our physicians are playing with very strong, lethal tools, the war they are waging produces costly fallout. Guess to whom? When a person plays with fire, somebody always gets burned, and that somebody is never the doctor.

Yet, we stay loyal because we honestly believe medical doctors will take better care of us in the long run. Well maybe that's not the case when we consider the risk.

Data from MyMedicalScore.com, titled by Medical Error Statistics (2020): "Deaths/Year & Malpractice Rates," reveals that medical errors cause an estimated 250,000 deaths in the United States annually. That total ranks third in the overall causes of death each year, following only heart disease and cancer, as initially cited in a Johns Hopkins study released in 2016. (50)

Continuing from the same study, "Death from medical errors could be even higher due to the way medical errors are often unreported on death certificates—with, some professionals estimating, as many as 440,000 people dying every year from medical mistakes." (50)

The study goes on to say, "These are not disease caused deaths—these are treatment caused deaths. Some sources like the CDC conveniently overlook medical errors as a cause of death and don't list them at all in their charts." (50) They are, however, documented through many other very reputable studies.

"Some categories for error include unnecessary surgeries, misdiagnoses, medication errors in a dosage prescribed or type of drug used, hospital errors, infections contracted in hospitals, deaths due to negative effects of drugs prescribed and believe it or not, patient misidentification." (50) Yes, the last one had enough incidents reported to make the list.

Do we expect the medical community to be human and make mistakes? Sure we do, but we also must acknowledge that the tools they use are not always as effective as we might hope and are very often lethal. For that reason alone, it's smart for patients to proceed with caution with this form of medical treatment since needless drugs, radiation, and surgeries can possibly cause irreparable damage. It should also give us the courage to seek second opinions, consider other options, and listen to our own good judgment in the process of deciding what medical treatment makes sense for us.

Still, in the face of facts like these, our medical community often remains arrogant and dismissive of alternative options. Although there are isolated physicians who absolutely won't acknowledge any form of alternative care, some younger physicians are more open and allow patients to talk freely about alternative methods they are using, and some even encourage complementary options. A caution remains that if you're seeking the approval from a medical doctor in advance of any alternative method or therapy, odds are the response will be negative or cool. For the most part, I believe medical physicians are still threatened by the overwhelming trend toward alternatives in which they have not been trained and over which they have no control.

Your doctor always knows best.

Your doctor may be very well trained and know a lot about his or her specialty, even general conventional practice, but that physician knows little about the overall health or healing of an individual patient. They don't know about the intricacies of how your specific body functions or the lifestyle you lead. They also know very little about preventive care, natural options, or even why or how some alternative modalities work.

Medical physicians are inadequately trained in any of the mind-body-spirit related disciplines. Is that important? you ask. Well, when it comes to nutrition, for example, there is a direct relationship with how very specific and nuanced nutritional recommendations can prevent or minimize the risk of heart disease, obesity, and allergies, just for three examples. At best medical physicians might only have a broad understanding.

When you calculate all the hours medical students spend during a minimum of a twelve-year education after high school in preparation to become a licensed physician, it's a big number. Yet, doctors only receive an average of 19.6 hours of nutritional training. (51) What they do know about diet and exercise merely scratches the surface of what would really make a difference for the patient.

To the myth again. Your doctors might know best about some things, but those same providers don't know very much about anything outside of drug therapy, related surgeries, or to which specialist you should be referred. The drug focus is a given when we analyze how dominant the pharmaceutical industry is in physician education and training.

Until recently, US pharmaceutical companies funded most US medical schools with very little regulation. In 2013, the American Medical Student Association released its PharmFree Scorecard, which continues to encourage medical schools to improve their policies on conflicts of interest and interactions with the pharmaceutical industry. They hope patients will have no doubt that decisions about care are based on science and a patient's best interests, not the marketing strategies of Big Pharma. This study has been conducted for six years as of 2013 with 73 percent of the 158 US medical schools now receiving an aggregate grade of A or B for their policies. That's compared to 102 last year and just 45 in 2009. (52)

I ask readers to think back to when their doctor graduated medical school. I'll bet it was more than ten years ago—so imagine what the conflict-of-interest grades might have been then. When massive funding exists, it's hard to avoid undue influence.

Always seek conventional medicine first.

Granted, going to your medical physician for the diagnosis of a complex issue makes total sense, so you know what you're dealing with. Staying with them in the early treatment stages is debatable. What makes no sense at all is running to the doctor for minor issues when you know what's wrong with you. At least, that's my opinion. I believe calling your doctor for a quick fix is more of a habit than a necessity and could be less healthy in the long run.

The question remains: How much better might a patient do healthwise if preventive measures or more natural options were enlisted before any condition became too bad? There's no doubt that the training medical physicians receive is slanted toward treatment over prevention, and sometimes initial treatment is aggressive. So, the question remains, does holding such a belief help you or harm you?

The overall reputation of the industry has already been put into question with the US longevity statistics—therefore, maybe it's time to look at conventional medicine specialty by specialty.

Someone with a very candid opinion about all of that is Andrew Weil, MD, who received his medical degree at Harvard and is an articulate and authoritative voice for alternative healing. Weil acknowledges that allopathic medicine does not always have all the answers.

In one of his earliest books titled *Spontaneous Healing*, and one of my favorites, Dr. Weil courageously and objectively lists what you can expect from conventional medicine and what you cannot. The *can* list includes managing trauma better than any other system of medicine, diagnosing and treating medical and surgical emergencies, treating acute bacterial infections with antibiotics, treating some parasitic and fungal infections, preventing many infectious diseases by immunization, diagnosing complex medical problems, replacing damaged hips and knees, getting good results with cosmetic and reconstructive surgery, and diagnosing and correcting hormonal deficiencies. (53)

He continues that allopathic medicine *cannot* adequately treat viral infections, cure most chronic degenerative diseases, effectively manage most kinds of mental illness, cure most forms of allergy or autoimmune disease, effectively manage psychosomatic illnesses, or cure most forms of cancer. Most objective physicians would agree with this list.

I have a couple of exceptions, from my own experience, regarding how well they correct hormonal deficiencies without harm and diagnose complex conditions that stem from stress or Candida Albicans, for example, both of which present a wide range of unrelated symptoms. In addition, physicians rarely acknowledge Candida as an issue because people always have that fungus in their system. What physicians forget to consider is not if a patient has it but how much they have. At some point Candida can become invasive to organs and to the immune function if not stopped when it grows out of control.

Other than those, I believe Dr. Weil's list is right on the money. Medical practitioners are willing to admit their vulnerability regarding certain conditions and illnesses but do so among themselves. That dialogue never extends to include their patient being privy to the facts.

Totally believe what your doctor tells you.

When you visit with your doctor, there are usually three bits of information he or she will impart: a diagnosis, a recommended treatment protocol, and a prognosis. Over the years, my experience has taught me to always believe the first, listen intently to the second—then decide independently what to do, and totally ignore the third. With that philosophy, I've done remarkably well over the last forty years. This is the reason for my point of view about the most potentially abusive of those three categories of advice, the prognosis.

The worst thing our medical practitioners do is to program our defeat. Many do that when delivering the prognosis of a condition. When a doctor tells you that you will have to live with a condition forever or that you might not live very long at all—it has impact. When words like that are spoken, something very powerful occurs. If you believe what is said, it zaps you of any remaining control and strength, robs you of your self-confidence, and creates a placebo-in-reverse effect. Yes, a powerful and damaging dynamic is created by physicians who overstep their field of knowledge by attempting to fortune-tell a patient's future.

Doctors don't realize the damage they can do. Again, it's not so much in delivering the diagnosis where they run into a problem, but rather how they deliver the prognosis. Patients are too often told, "There is no cure for this condition." "All we can do is treat the symptoms—the condition will not go away." "You will just have to live with it." "There is nothing more that can be done." Or even more shocking, "You only have (so many) months to live."

There are other, more truthful options. It's perfectly fine for doctors to deliver their interpretation of fact, but they should do so with hope and with honesty. Simply adding the caveat that the patient "doesn't have to be one of the statistics" is not being dishonest, instead it keeps hope alive. A physician would be even more truthful if he or she said, "We don't have a good track record with this disease, or our odds offer only a 50 percent survival rate. But you don't have to be one of those statistics, you can look elsewhere." Or, they could simply say, "*I* am not able to help you, however, help could still exist. You should try another form of treatment." That is not only keeping hope alive but also telling the truth.

When a patient who is vulnerable and who is already fearful of a bad diagnosis hears a prognosis of doom, it can become a self-fulfilling prophecy, or worse, it can become a hex. We have all heard of the placebo response, with patients showing improvement if they simply believe they are taking something that will help them. Well, that same response can work in reverse. People can believe there is no hope if that message is delivered by someone they trust. The power of the mind is astounding.

According to Dr. Howard Brody, coauthor of *The Placebo Response* and professor of family medicine and philosophy at Michigan State University, a positive placebo response occurs when three factors are optimally present: the meaning of the illness experience for the patient is altered in a positive manner, the patient is supported by a caring group, and the patient's sense of mastery and control over the illness is enhanced. It also became clear that a physician can strip a patient of two or three of these factors with a poorly worded prognosis.

If a physician has made an absolute statement with the medical diagnosis or prognosis to you without offering any hope at all, a behavioral command has been established. This then becomes the predominant mindset for everyone surrounding you. You believe it, your doctor believes it, all who treat you believe it, and your family and friends believe it, so therefore, that is precisely what happens.

Sometimes your doctor doesn't have to say anything at all except name the disease. Even today, uttering the diagnosis of HIV/AIDS and even some forms of cancer can terrify a patient. Yet there are so many patients in the world who have totally recovered from stage-four cancers, and even advanced cases of HIV/AIDS, without killing themselves first with the drugs prescribed. Some people look outside of conventional medical care, and some find results.

With a prognosis that is deemed chronic or even terminal by a physician, I suggest patients accept such labels as the physician's opinion only and not the final word. The fact exists that scientific-based allopathic medicine has no known cure for many conditions, and many patients just look past that fact allowing themselves to be further poked, prodded, and dosed with chemotherapy in Hail Mary efforts with little expectation for success. They then live the rest of their short lives without any quality of life at all.

In my case, the prognoses ended up always being wrong. So, I hope that more people will not blindly accept the scientific, medical model and reach out occasionally to see if hope exists through other methods. Or you can believe the prognosis, expect to die, and that will eventually be the case.

If you can't prove it scientifically, it isn't valid.

Another belief that may not hold water is that everything must be proven scientifically to be credible. When dismissing alternative care, conventional medicine likes to use that provider's lack of results from clinical trials or double-blind studies as the rationale. That's a false comparison since alternative or holistic methods are not uniform in their practice and all elements are customized for each patient, therefore establishing "standards" is impossible. That doesn't mean this method is invalid, it just makes it different—but more importantly, the metrics used in scientific studies are not always perfect themselves.

Conventional medical physicians have been taught that if you can't measure it, it can't possibly work. Well, who can measure faith, for example? Who can measure personal responsibility? Who can measure diligence? Yet, all three make a huge difference in how well a person will eventually recover, and even though all three are relatively immeasurable by themselves, considered on the whole, they are extraordinarily powerful.

Here is where I have issues with scientific trials and studies in the first place. First, the fact that they look for a consistent group to test and then consider the results of that test valid is flawed in my mind since thinking any test group was consistently constructed in the first place is an invalid assumption. Besides the emotional, mental, and spiritual aspects of individual patients, let's just take the physical. Out of one hundred individuals chosen, no two are even close to being the same person. They have different body types, for example. Some are ectomorphs, others are endomorphs, and still others are mesomorphs. Those three body types don't function nearly the same—they may or may not store fat, may have more or less muscle mass, and may have other vulnerabilities or assets.

Additionally, some people have different chemical sensitivities than others, some are not truthful about their lifestyle when filling out the application (diet and alcohol, for example), stress levels aren't considered, and their genetic predispositions might dramatically differ. So, to ever claim uniformity truly is a non sequitur.

Another issue with scientific research is not only how the research is conducted but how it's reported. They routinely state the *average* of how many improved in the test, not the average amount of improvement for each patient. So, when we hear someone tell us that 80 percent of the patients taking XYZ drug improved, *wow*, it sounds impressive right? Wrong. Again, that doesn't mean the patients improved 80 percent—it means on average 80 percent of the total number of patients showed improvement. To be totally truthful, they should say that 80 percent of the patients showed *some* improvement—yet while never mentioning the degree of improvement, they also happen to leave out the word *some*, so we never know how much improvement patients may have realized. Was it 5 percent, 10 percent, 35 percent, or 70 percent? Nobody says, and if the rate of improvement isn't stated, odds are it was fairly low.

We also must remember that the remaining 20 percent showed no improvement at all. So, what happened to them? What percentage stayed the same and what percentage died from taking the XYZ drug? It would be one thing if the results of clinical trials were only deceiving in how they report improvements, but it's worse than that. Often, they avoid reporting deaths and serious injuries totally. Now that's a real oversight!

The NIH, the parent organization for the United States National Library of Medicine, in their published report on the haphazard reporting of deaths in clinical trials, states that in five hundred randomly selected from ClinicalTrials.gov records, only 15 percent of those records reported a number for deaths. They continue to detail how total deaths could be determined in some of the groups or subgroups of participants only 56 percent of the time and were discordant in 19 percent of the cases. In others, 48 percent showed no information on deaths, while 33 percent were discordant. There was much more detail in the results, but the conclusions were unambiguous. Deaths are variably reported in ClinicalTrials.gov records. A reliable total from each group or subgroup of participants cannot always be determined with any certainty or can be discordant with numbers reported in corresponding trial publications. (55)

I can't let this drop here because conventional medicine has unfoundedly discounted alternative methodology for decades, so it's time they are also held accountable. It's fair to question the scientific proof argument—if for no other reason than because of this article that appeared on August 23, 2022, in *Natural News.*

"Former The British Medical Journal (BMJ) editor Richard Smith penned an opinion piece for the journal suggesting that health research has become so corrupted and untrustworthy that people should just assume it is fraudulent and false until proven otherwise." (55)

From the same piece, "Smith's article reveals how research fraud is a systemic problem that dates back decades—and is only getting worse." He continued, "The trials were all published in prestigious neurosurgery journals and had multiple co-authors," Smith explained. "None of the co-authors had contributed patients to the trials and some didn't know that they were co-authors until after the trials were published."

Do we truly believe pharmaceutical companies will not manipulate the data to suit their purposes of quick approval or to gain approval in the first place? We all know the answer to that. So, if the requirement for the validity of anecdotal evidence obtained through more natural means is scientific proof, their point is ridiculous.

Can anecdotal results from holistic or alternative methods be taken seriously?

Although everyone might acknowledge that it's not possible to measure holistic healing with scientifically based measurement tools, one still must acknowledge that successes do occur.

There are books everywhere from very credible medical doctors who have become more enlightened and expanded in their practices to include other methods of care than the conventional allopathic model. Some of these doctors focus on the healing power of prayer, of love, and of visualization and affirmations as well as Ayurvedic medicine, traditional Chinese medicine, and so many more. Each is filled with case studies and examples of remarkable results using methods not measurable by any scientific standard. Additionally, there are hundreds of books by authors who have recovered from conditions or diseases that seemed unlikely or impossible. Still other books exist by alternative providers who want to share therapies or methods that have brought complete healing to their patients. In those cases, they always include examples or case studies for reinforcement.

So, results in this field, although considered anecdotal, are available anywhere you'd want to look. I happen to be a perfect example since I've demonstrated anecdotal success at least seven different times over the last forty years. In all cases, with me specifically, I used a holistic care model and considered every aspect of my being in the healing process. Mine was a comprehensive approach, to be sure.

Conventional medical doctors don't have time for comprehensive, holistic approaches to care. Their practices are more tightly scheduled, allowing them only to glance at a chart before entering the room, chat for a few minutes with the patient, and focus on the symptom, and their efforts generally end with a little advice, a new prescription, or booking an appointment for more tests or some procedure. Pretty simple, really. I just happen to believe that the most lasting and effective solutions are always comprehensive approaches influenced by an abundance of factors. Comparing the two is like comparing a solo flute to an orchestra.

Still, even though conventional medicine will acknowledge that many of the elements of holistic healing or even alternative approaches are valid, such as belief system, lifestyle habits, stress levels, and even prayer as well as a handful of methods like acupuncture and a couple more, they still don't bestow on them the same level of importance as drug therapy, radiation, or surgery, alone.

I guess I am just a different breed of person and prefer to receive treatment from people who will let me participate in my care, provide a customized program based on my input, and protect my body from damage by using harmless therapies. Granted, my results might not be statistically valid, but I'm perfectly content having merely been a successful anecdote, over and over again.

Chapter 6
GETTING WELL—
NOTHING IS IMPOSSIBLE

I was a devoted conventional medical patient in my early adult life. I knew who to listen to, who I trusted, and my personal belief system had long been established. I was an accomplished woman and assumed I was well informed, exposed, and savvy. I was good to go until I reached my late thirties. Then I wasn't.

The turning point for me occurred in 1981, when the way I had led my life finally caught up to me. I was thirty-seven years old and had been running on a treadmill for the past eight years, and the treadmill was winning.

People find themselves in routines they don't even notice. One day just leads to another, and the same habits continue. That was the case with me. I pushed my body, pushed my body, and continued to push. I didn't think I was doing anything wrong; I had a lot on my plate and the more responsibility I assumed, the more I worked. At some point, something had to give. In my case, it was my body.

As you will see, once my first serious illness hit, I tried to stay committed to conventional medicine, as I always had, but finally couldn't any longer. It always takes something to be the trigger for change, and for me it was seeing the rapid deterioration of my health when I wasn't even forty years old.

When the light finally went on, as happens with many, some delicately make a shift, but I was different since I jumped feet first into an entirely new life. I didn't hesitate, I as was fearless, since being old and decrepit at my age wasn't in the program. The move I made was instinctive, not intellectual—which I believe in hindsight is always best.

Anyway, I'm not advocating for other people to take the plunge like I did. Instead, most will simply dip their toe in the water and continue dipping until they're comfortable enough to wade in knee high and then waist deep to find better answers toward a healthy life.

I was just sick of being sick. Other people might be tired of taking countless prescriptions, still others might resent when a doctor tells them they're just getting older—when they look around and find people even older than they are who are much more healthy and vital. When you've finally had enough and decide it's time for something different, this is the book for you. You may not end up bolting, but I promise you—you'll feel more empowered.

My journey to recovering from one serious condition after another and then another didn't just happen one day. Nothing ever happens that easily. To get to the fascinating part of my story, let me present the backstory first.

How everything started.

I grew up only being familiar with conventional medical care. I didn't know anything about the alternative world and didn't care. I was raised a meat-and-potatoes kind of girl in a small town in the Midwest. I think I was also a little scrawny and not too healthy since I seem to remember catching colds more often than my friends.

As a woman in my twenties, I always had allergies, so I got allergy shots. I also routinely developed upper respiratory issues during that period, so I was prescribed antihistamines, decongestants, and a drug called theophylline to open my respiratory tubes. I took them all daily. Antibiotics and steroids were prescribed, too, but more intermittently.

When I took the theophylline capsule first thing in the morning, it gave me the energy I needed to pull myself out of bed since I worked so hard and was likely very run-down. I took this drug for years, which I don't believe was particularly healthy, because many decades later,

I realized it produced an amphetamine-like effect, which just made it easier for me to push my body even harder. I might as well have been on speed since, although more addictive and a little stronger, amphetamines are amphetamines. Everything I ever took was prescribed to me by highly credible pulmonologists in Phoenix, and I was prescribed lots of drugs.

Once I opened my own business at twenty-eight, I was way over my skis. I was the sole owner of the company, and the pressure of sustaining an undercapitalized, fast-growing advertising and public relations agency kept me continually stressed. I took no vacation for eight years and was making a multitude of other lousy lifestyle choices at the time such as smoking cigarettes, self-medicating with alcohol, and as a single parent, trying to find time to date and eventually marrying someone who was emotionally abusive. Top it all off, my industry was one of the most high-pressure around with constant deadlines and the need to produce results for dozens of clients on a constant basis.

I was also overcommitted. By this time, I had also become a community leader and served on multiple nonprofit boards all while trying to be a great mom to my beloved son, a good wife, and a dutiful daughter to ailing parents. Everything eventually took its toll, and my body gave out.

Rheumatoid arthritis.

One night in 1981, I was wakened at three o'clock in the morning with excruciating pain in my right knee. I was immobilized for hours, unable to twist my leg or move the muscle that regulated the knee. The pain was unbelievable—if I even twitched that leg, the sharp pain was nearly unbearable. I thought my cartilage had dislodged.

The next day after the pain released enough for me to move a little, my husband took me to my chiropractor who checked my knee for something out of place; everything seemed fine. Eventually all the pain subsided, and I went back to my life.

Weeks later a similar attack occurred with my left hip—also in the middle of the night. This time, I had to be carried into my doctor's office because standing vertically, which put weight on that hip, generated unbearable pain once again. I was immediately referred to a rheumatologist. The diagnosis from him was palindromic rheumatism, a rare type of inflammatory arthritis characterized by recurrent, self-resolving inflammatory attacks occurring in and around the joints. It is most common with people between the ages of twenty and fifty.

I was told these attacks would become less frequent and less severe, and that for many patients, it eventually transitioned into rheumatoid arthritis. He was right. Some months later after a rash of similar attacks that eventually became more frequent—just as severe but less jolting and longer in duration—I was back in his office, a victim of rheumatoid arthritis (RA).

As someone with RA, the expected degenerative, debilitating symptoms plagued me, but in my case, they seemed to have come on all too quickly and with a complete vengeance. I was told this disease was incurable, or *chronic* was the word they liked to use. Anyway, this rheumatologist hoped to be able to minimize the symptoms with medication. He was the best in town, and I trusted him implicitly.

After eighteen months of conventional medical treatment, powerful anti-inflammatory drugs, and routine trips to the emergency room for steroid injections, my physician decided to prescribe a form of chemotherapy called methotrexate to quiet my T-cells, calm down my immune system, and thereby mitigate the increasingly painful symptoms. Sitting in his office at the time, the last year and a half flashed before my eyes.

It was apparent to me that I was not really improving. Even with all the drugs I was being given, energy-wise I could only function six hours a day at work (50 percent for me) before I returned home, collapsed on the sofa for the rest of the evening, and had to be helped into the bathroom or bedroom by my twelve-year-old son or my husband because my joints continued to stiffen up in the evening. Deformity had already started in my hands, and the swelling, stiffness, and pain were unrelenting in nearly every joint in my body. I had lost nearly 20 percent of my hair, and my skin looked like a woman in her seventies (I was half that then). My body was aging so rapidly I could hardly believe it. This, I thought, was not the way I wanted to live.

It was then I realized that taking methotrexate was simply adding one drug more. This time, as a chemotherapy agent and immune system suppressant, methotrexate wasn't a benign drug. It required routine liver testing during use, and since RA was a "chronic" condition, I could expect to be taking that drug for the rest of my life. That's when I decided I wasn't getting better, my meds were just getting stronger—a very bad trend.

That's when I also quit the conventional medical approach to RA and took matters into my own hands. I had no idea where I was going or what I was going to do, but I knew it wasn't the current path. I'd had it with rheumatologists and the conventional medical "experts."

Somewhere in the back of my mind, I knew answers existed for everything, if people just took time to look. I honestly believed people who never found answers to their issues couldn't because they always quit too soon. Knowing answers existed somewhere, I guess I subconsciously turned it over. I didn't talk to God or even ask for His help, but somebody heard me. Without doing research or trying to figure out what could be done that conventional medicine couldn't do, I just opened up and was willing to be led. Then, in total ignorance, the first step in my holistic healing journey began.

After my husband mentioned how worried he was about me to a friend, that friend recommended a very credible nutritionist in town. I was given the nutritionist's name—it was Dee Kell—and I called her. Answers were coming to me, and I was totally receptive. From Mrs. Kell, who died many years ago, I learned more about the power of the immune system, what all pharmaceuticals did to compromise our immune systems, and how to start looking at the whole of my body and my life, which were all playing roles in my illness.

Without prompting, I went off all medications within months, so my immune system could begin to recover without interference and learn to again function healthily. I began a healing journey that led to marked improvement within the first ninety days. It began with Mrs. Kell, but throughout the time I saw her, other helpers were also brought my way. Of course, I used her nutritional therapy, learned to control my systemic candidiasis, and added several supplements—which initially were also credited to her. I then made significant lifestyle and attitude changes and got more rest—within two to three years, my immune system was strong enough to fight the disease and win. No drugs, no doctors, no disfigurement, and no symptoms. Today I am as flexible and graceful as a dancer and look many years younger.

I'll provide a few more details as to the emotional/mental and spiritual elements of healing from this condition as well as others as we continue. The overviews that follow are meant only to give you the big picture of what I did.

Psoriasis.

One day, during my RA healing journey, my legs began to itch. I thought it was dry skin, but I could feel hardening under the surface, and lotions didn't help. The more I scratched, the more the skin became irritated, and soon I noticed dry, red, scaly patches appearing. When I scratched them, they bled. It was psoriasis, and it was ugly and terribly difficult to deal with because the itching never seemed to stop.

Ironically, for me, this condition ran from just under my knees to my ankles on both legs. I was given topical creams, but the more I read about the condition and the prognosis, the more discouraged I became. Of course, my doctors didn't seem to have a cure at the time, and back then, dermatologists may not have realized psoriasis was tied to the immune system, so they didn't offer immune suppressant drugs, which I wouldn't have taken anyway. Back then, there was also a national association I could join to commiserate with others sharing the same issue. My legs looked horrible, and for more than two years, I only wore slacks.

Once again, I became discouraged with the answers I received from my doctors, so I just applied the cream I was given. "If that doesn't work," one doctor said, "we'll try a different cream." It seemed to me the itching was a symptom of something much deeper, but the doctors were unconcerned about digging further. So, again I walked away, this time from any medical opinion or treatment dealing with psoriasis

You'll soon see a pattern emerging in my life, where with condition after condition, I'd give scientific medicine a chance to help me, and time and time again, they'd disappoint—their only answers being one drug and then another. Eventually, the bulk of my care became alternatively sourced and self-directed using my body as my compass. More detail will follow.

Back to the psoriasis. Once I discontinued all the prescription drugs I had been taking, so my body's immune system could recover from the RA and begin to function on its own again, I noticed something else happening. The psoriasis began to disappear too. As my immune system grew stronger and the drugs and toxins were out of my system, the condition totally disappeared. Emotional work also helped. I have been psoriasis-free for thirty-five years. My legs returned to normal quickly.

Chronic respiratory issues and allergies.

As I mentioned earlier, from the time I was in my mid-twenties for nearly ten years I was plagued by chronic allergies and upper respiratory issues. Colds and more colds, which generally settled in my chest, routinely resulted in bronchitis, pneumonia, or terrible colds that dragged on for what seemed like forever. I ran to the pulmonary specialist routinely and took antihistamines and bronchial drugs daily and antibiotics at least every month. When my cold or flu symptoms got too bad, I was given steroids to make it possible for me to keep working. As a single mom with a new business, I could never afford to be sick.

When the rheumatoid arthritis hit a few years later, I was still battling the respiratory symptoms. Then as I began the holistic healing journey, gradually eliminated all my prescription medicines, and began the process of allowing my immune system to become stronger on its own, everything improved. By the time my arthritis and psoriasis were gone, so were my allergies.

Today, the chronic respiratory issues are history. Once or twice a year I'd catch a cold when my grandchildren were young, but the preventive therapies I learned about generally stopped the process before it progressed into any full-blown condition. Even if I come down with a cold today, it barely gets a foothold since I know what to do to stop it; therefore, my chest and lungs are never affected.

Today, I am so much healthier overall due to the natural antiviral vitamins and supplements I discovered along the way. That is how I learned to maintain my good health even through several epidemics or pandemics that occurred from 1990 until today. Once my body was back in charge, my life totally changed.

Leukemia (the first time).

Tired, I was so tired, but being a bit of a workaholic and the fact that I had just finished cochairing a political fundraiser in Phoenix for a presidential candidate on top of running my business, I just chalked the fatigue up to overwork and overcommitment. Over the next several weeks, I grew weaker, and neither rest nor sleep seemed to help me rebound. My energy level was in the basement, so I decided to go to my holistic physician, who also happened to be an MD, for a routine physical three months later. That was in late August 1999.

A day or so later, I received a phone call at home from my doctor telling me my white count looked high and that she'd like to have me come back for more blood work. I did, and a couple of days later, she called again to tell me she was very concerned and recommended I see a hematologist.

I asked her, "Why—what's the matter?"

"You may have lymphoma or leukemia. You really need to see a specialist," she said.

My doctor tried to break the news without overdramatizing the whole thing, but there was no question, she was making a firm suggestion.

I'm a tough cookie; I handle stress well and am usually the strong one in the face of any crisis, but I will tell you her last comment brought me to my knees. I was in shock. I had spent years getting over the rheumatoid arthritis, psoriasis, and chronic allergies. I just couldn't understand why this was happening to me now.

For the next several hours I walked around the house in a fog, and when I gained enough clarity, I'd pick up a book and read about the various forms of lymphoma and leukemia to try to relate to the symptoms. When my husband came home that evening, I was sitting on the floor, my knees to my chest, with a book of symptoms cradled in my arms. I hadn't moved from the small downstairs office that was adjacent to the kitchen. I had used that room for collecting healing stones, various self-help books, and medical books, and it was located to the right of the back door where we always entered from the back patio. I was staring straight ahead. My husband knew instantly something was terribly wrong. He sat down next to me. I said nothing for a few minutes and then I told him.

After allowing myself to wallow in pity for a few days (yes, that's completely normal) after receiving the initial news, I began massive oral doses of vitamin C (increased gradually) on my own and had started emotional therapy using a book by Louise Hay and another by Caroline Myss to guide me.

It took nearly a month after my bone marrow biopsy to receive the final diagnosis of LGL leukemia, large granular lymphocytic leukemia, an uncommon form of chronic leukemia. The diagnosis came from the University of Arizona Cancer Center in Tucson. This was a chronic condition that was expected to be ongoing unless my white count escalated and it became acute, which could happen if my immune system became any weaker. That was the reason they monitored my blood work every three months. Chemotherapy, the same drug as for the RA, so again I rejected it because I was committed to the vitamin C therapy.

As allopathic doctors began to routinely monitor me every three months, I felt that was inadequate since my care was self-directed, so I had a holistic MD order my blood draws every two weeks so I could chart my ongoing results. I watched the white count and lymph count (the two distinct markers for this condition) and recorded them on a graph while I continued high oral doses of vitamin C daily and IVs of vitamin C weekly. Toward the end, I did some emotional healing work, which accelerated everything.

By the time I visited the doctors again, my blood work had stabilized. Over time, the oncologists in Tucson, who had watched my progress as my white count and lymph count gradually declined, finally saw the results. Twenty months later both markers were perfectly normal, and I was well. I stayed perfectly healthy through the publication of my first book, *Get Well: Even When You've Been Told You Can't* (2008), and even beyond.

Hyperthyroidism.

During the leukemia diagnosis, I began seeing a thickening in my neck—like a goiter appearing. I had noticed it in photos and thought I'd go once again to my holistic MD for her opinion. She sent me to an endocrinologist since I had a few other symptoms as well. I was diagnosed with hyperthyroidism, a condition that over time can produce a goiter in the neck, irritability, heat intolerance, increased sweating, protruding eyes, and often tachycardia. They thought it was Graves' disease.

After the initial visit with this endocrinologist and her analysis of the results of my blood work, she was very eager to prescribe a drastic but common treatment, which was to blow out my thyroid—no, that's not the medical description. She asked me to undergo a procedure that consisted of giving me an IV injection containing radioactive iodine, which would render my thyroid inactive. Thereafter, I'd be taking a medication every day to replace the thyroxine that my thyroid normally produced. I was not excited about putting radioactive anything into my bloodstream while currently living with leukemia, a cancer of the blood—so I questioned that. The doctor remained unfazed.

She wanted this procedure done right away—by the following week. She said I would be at great risk of this condition affecting my heart if I didn't act quickly. The endocrinologist also assured me the treatment was harmless—yet in the same breath she stated that I couldn't be around children or pregnant women for forty-eight hours or share eating utensils with anyone else during that time. The radioactive iodine I had taken could affect them too. So much for harmless!

She was way too urgent in pressing me to undergo this very serious protocol, so I asked her how long it would take for my heart to eventually become affected. She cautioned me that within a couple of years that could happen. *Well*, I thought, *that isn't next Thursday.*

I politely made the appointment that day for the procedure the following week, so as not to make a scene, but the next day called her receptionist and canceled it. As you might guess, I took matters into my own hands and asked a brilliant alternative cancer research guy in Wichita, Kansas, whom I'd met a month or two before (there are no coincidences) for his recommendation. I asked him if he were diagnosed with hyperthyroidism, what steps would he take?

He told me that for some people this condition indicates a deficiency in iodine. Now that might sound strange since iodine is in our salt, but whether that type of iodine is absorbed by the person's body or not is another issue. He said there was an at-home diagnostic tool and very specific treatment protocol that might work. Of course, I tried it and within ten hours I knew my answer. I was iodine deficient, but the result of applying a specific size tincture of iodine on one forearm to first determine the deficiency and then to cure it was that there was no longer a need for further treatment. The next time I went to the doctor, a couple of weeks later, I was diagnosed with hypothyroidism—exactly the opposite!

One more time, answers were found for every one of the conditions I faced outside of conventional medicine and without pharmaceutical drugs—each using methods that were harmless and were counter to any treatments scientific medicine offered. Everything I did made my body stronger!

One lengthy journey ended, but there was one more to go.

Chapter 7
GETTING WELL, AGAIN—
STILL NOT IMPOSSIBLE

Perfect health doesn't go on forever, especially if we slide back into destructive lifestyle choices and habits. That's what happened to me. I had jumped into another stellar romantic relationship, and this one drained me energy-wise making it easy to ignore my old routine and the positive lifestyle choices I'd adopted.

To keep ourselves healthy, we must routinely take inventory of our bodies—how our bodies feel and react—and if little things go awry, we're on top of the situation and can fix them or maybe readjust our routine. We know when adjustments need to be made when our metabolism slows down, when we're under more stress than usual, or our weight has done more than creep up over time. We notice those signals, and whether we make corrections to our normal routine or not doesn't matter if we're paying attention to our bodies. Eventually, we all decide to tweak something here and there.

Well, I forgot to notice, so of course I forgot to tweak. In fact, I was so distracted, I was transported back decades to a time when I pushed my body again and again—like I did when I was working eighty hours a week. This time, unfortunately, I was in my mid-sixties. With my new relationship, I was walking two or more miles a day, very actively dancing late into the evening, running up and down stairs in my friend's two-story condo, and getting much less than my normal nine hours of sleep a night, which my body needed. There were a couple of other factors at play too.

I really had no time to rest, but life was so stimulating and fun that I pushed through it. We even hiked into the mountains of New Mexico and camped with miners because my friend was doing some sort of mineral research. When I did take time for physical rest, it was only to write any one of a series of business plans for mining ventures and a proposed mass transit system in Florida, which we both flew back to present. The pressure of writing and producing business documents was my downtime. Trust me, I was extraordinarily active for over six decades of life. Over two years, it began to show.

Am I blaming the guy I was dating? Not at all, I was just stupid, and yes, lapses of good judgment can happen to very smart people. I took my good health for granted and stretched the boundaries I had previously established. It was all my fault as illness always is—if we dig down deep enough.

There were several other reasons for my energy decline over this period, in addition to those I already cited, since I later discovered this man was an energy vampire and I was around him 24/7 for over two years. That was one of the two worst issues. Ask any massage therapist or person who works with the human body, and they'll confirm that energy vampires exist and are deadly. They slowly and consistently rob another person of energy, and over time, there isn't much left for the victim.

The other was the consistent lack of my required level of sleep. That one I won't explain.

CMV, rheumatoid arthritis, and leukemia, once again.

I gradually became very run-down and susceptible to a massive cytomegalovirus (CMV) infection, which I eventually developed. That CMV must have been hiding in my body for more than fifty years. Eventually the virus exploded in my system and compromised my immune system to the point where my rheumatoid arthritis returned, and so did my leukemia. I ended up with all three major illnesses at the same time, and it seemed to take forever to fully recover.

To explain the virus, CMV is a common virus, and once infected, the body retains it for life. This virus can lie dormant for years and flare up when the person is particularly vulnerable. I was certainly that. The virus itself is related to the viruses that cause chickenpox, which I had as a child, and herpes simplex, which is cold sores, which I also had when I was younger. It is also related to Epstein-Barr and mononucleosis, neither of which were ever formally identified in me, but I had many of those symptoms during my first health crisis in the '80s. One thing I learned was that people with weakened immune systems who get CMV have more serious symptoms, and for some, it can become fatal. My case was particularly challenging.

The CMV had eventually grown to such proportions that the levels were four times higher than anything any of my doctors had ever seen. It seems people can exist with that virus in their systems at a count of one hundred or lower without an active disease. My doctors had seen a viral load count of four or five hundred in serious cases prior, but after testing, mine was over two thousand. A count from two to five thousand signals the development of end organ disease. (56)

My immune system was overwhelmed, and it is no wonder the RA and the leukemia came back. I could barely function, cried often from exhaustion, and my physicians referred to my emotional reaction as being completely battle weary. I was one sick girl, who was sixty-six years old at the time.

With this new virus and the other two issues occurring simultaneously, my body was unable to fight them all at once, so I broke from my standard rejection of pharmaceutical drugs and took a mild antiviral drug some people take consistently for a different prophylactic reason. For me it was to help lighten that massive viral load before my heart, lungs, or kidneys became permanently weakened. I took that drug for one year, which provided enough relief to give my body the flexibility it needed to fight the RA and leukemia with natural help.

So, you see, I'm not one to totally shun conventional medicine; I'm smart enough to use it when there are no other options. I was grateful for the additional antiviral support. Side note: I also believe my body responded more quickly to the drug I was given because taking any drug is such a rarity for me.

I hope readers will note that I have never said conventional medicine is horrible and to never use it. In the case of emergencies or if an illness is so severe you might not have long to live, do whatever you have to do to put your finger in the dike while you are filling your body's reservoir with natural treatments to keep your body strong throughout the process, which is what I did, and it was smart.

For the rheumatoid arthritis, I reinstated my earlier strategy to re-strengthen my immune system, and eventually that program returned it to good working order, so it would stop the autoimmune reaction that attacked my joints. Yes, I went back to my healthy lifestyle with lots of sleep, a proper diet, absolutely no alcohol (during healing), and supple-mentation that made sense at the time. I also replenished my energy with solitude (which works for me) and practiced living in loving emotions, total forgiveness, and more gratitude. More about immune strengthen-ing specifics coming up in a future chapter.

For the leukemia, you guessed it—back to massive doses of vitamin C both intravenously and orally. I was in bed for two-and-a-half years, but not bedridden. Since I lived alone—yes, that boyfriend was gone—I still cooked my meals, bought my groceries, drove myself to the doctor, and managed to function a tiny bit at a time. The way it worked was I'd muster up energy to walk into the kitchen and sit in a chair I had there to rest. Then I'd stand to fix something to eat and intermittently sit and rest while the food was being prepared. Then, I'd take the food back to bed and would eat while my body totally rested. Rinse and repeat throughout the day. I sat and rested a lot regardless of what I was doing. Many days, I slept most of the day to rest for another outing of a couple of hours the next day. It's amazing how we manage to function when there isn't another option.

I was unable to do consulting work for another two years, and although by then I was a more mobile, I still had little or no energy, which potential clients could clearly recognize. The years without work and the cost of medical care, not covered by insurance, drained me of the rest of my financial resources—the balance that was left from a costly divorce ten years prior. The additional stress from the financial pressure didn't help.

This story is not to make readers feel sorry for me; on the contrary, it's to further prove that even living under some of the most stressful conditions—since I also had to downsize once again during this period and did so by myself—one can still recover. I needn't remind anyone how exhausting it is to pack and move a good size residence, and doing that alone took me weeks. Still, with all of that going on in my life, I ended up victorious over disease. Nothing, dear readers, is impossible.

Thankfully, after about eighteen months the viral condition was the first to disappear, then the RA, and the leukemia took the longest. Nothing with me ever seemed to be easy, but it's amazing what a person can overcome when remaining ill is not on one's agenda. I still wasn't well when the next thing hit.

Finally, neutropenia.

This one was a big surprise. It had now been over six years of recovering from the other three conditions, and my immune system had been taxed to the limit. I was nearly through the end of the leukemia journey when I began to develop another condition. This one was neutropenia. That's another bad one. Strangely, a person doesn't really realize when it is developing, except for the lack of energy, but since I had been living with very little energy for the last six years, I guess I didn't notice that contributor.

Neutropenia is a condition where lower-than-normal levels of neutrophils exist in a person's blood. A neutrophil is a type of white blood cell that one's bone marrow primarily makes to fight infections in the body and destroy germs that cause those infections, like viruses and bacteria. Luckily for me, as a habit from my last bout with illness, I always kept a record of my blood work so I could track the appropriate markers. I also kept copies of the complete blood count (CBC) reports. Those reports and my tracking always showed me trend lines on how well I was doing with my healing. Thankfully, I also had a holistic MD who placed a standing order for my blood work every two weeks—so I now could track my neutrophil count.

This irregularity, the neutropenia, was caught by one of the allopathic physicians on my team, who just monitored my progress in the event I ever got worse. He was an oncologist, explained neutropenia to me, and cautioned me about ever contracting a bacteria or virus while levels were low. It seemed anything I caught might kill me. The bacterial infections were less risky since I'd immediately get a high fever as the bacteria spread unchecked, and recognizing that, I could go quickly to an emergency room where I'd receive massive IV antibiotics once they became aware of my condition (I had records, remember?). That kind of infection could perhaps be stopped.

Contracting a virus was a totally different situation. Since it always takes too long to identify what type of virus a person has and then find the appropriate antiviral, if one even existed, there wouldn't be time. With no immunity, that virus would spread through my body like wildfire with no internal mechanism to contain it. I was obviously very careful.

I charted, watched, and when my neutrophil levels got into the danger zone, I'd put on a mask to protect against potential exposure outside of my home. I was living a COVID-19 protocol long before it was popular. I was even forbidden from shopping for fresh produce for fear I'd pick up some bug on the lettuce, an apple, or even scallions. My body would be unable to defend against any foreign invader. I lived like Bubble Boy, if you remember photos years ago of the little guy who had no immunity and lived in a plexiglass bubble. Then, from time to time, my neutrophil count would climb a bit and leave the danger zone. It was unpredictable and only identifiable with the blood work I had, now weekly. All I could do was rest, pray (asking for strength to do what He asked of me), eat well, and any emotional work that might make sense to maintain the health I had left.

My team of "observers" watched me, and of course my oncologist was now suggesting I take methotrexate (sound familiar?), the same chemotherapy drug that was recommended decades earlier for my RA, to suppress my T-cells (immune system). He was assuming I had autoimmune neutropenia because of my past RA history, and he was probably right. I still couldn't make myself take a chemical that was merely a Band-Aid fix. Besides, that drug, which required routine liver testing, produced side effects, and I'd be taking it the rest of my life. Forget any quality of life. I may have been exhausted with the neutropenia but otherwise was in pretty good shape. I understood all the benefits of methotrexate but couldn't totally acquiesce and eventually didn't have to.

By this time, the CMV was gone, my rheumatoid arthritis was gone, and my leukemia was really doing well but it had not yet disappeared, and the neutropenia was a becoming a challenge. What happened next might be called a miracle, but it wasn't. It was, once again, something being brought into my life on purpose—as it always is.

The final healing—a miracle?

Although much of my journey was miraculous because the body is just that—miraculous—my healing rituals more actively dealt with the physical and emotional or mental aspects of mind-body-spirit medicine. The spiritual piece, to this point, was covered with my trust and belief that in God's universe, answers do exist. I continued to trust that I'd be led and that faith was my strength. If I was meant to find answers, I'd find them, and if not, I'd pass knowing I'd done everything I was called to do. I could accept that.

This final step on this journey was a more active form of spiritual activity, one I had never really experienced before. It came by accident, although I know there are no accidents. What happened next some might consider totally bizarre or completely unbelievable.

Here's the story. My dearest friend, with whom I've been close for over thirty years, now lives out of the country, although she used to reside in Phoenix. Our relationship is more remote these days—especially since the coronavirus years impacted travel.

Over that thirty-year history, my clairaudient and clairvoyant gifts developed, and my friend's healing gifts showed up, quite by accident too. So, when I would develop a bad headache, I'd call her, and she'd help me on the phone. She was masterful at talking me through dissolving the headache pain. I don't think the methodology she used was something completely foreign in alternative circles, but she and I were particularly tuned in to each other. We both had intuitive gifts and could also give each other reinforcing guidance on life issues and even health. In other words, we'd both ask about things and receive answers.

A quick sidebar. After seven years of this last healing journey, the toll it had taken on my overall energy and the fact I wasn't getting any younger, I had accepted that if I was supposed to leave the planet, I'd be fine with that. I just wasn't one to lie down and die. I was sort of objective about the whole thing and not emotionally attached since I knew life came with a round trip ticket—we just weren't privy to the return date we were given.

At this point, I was about seventy-two years of age and had lived a remarkable life! I looked great for all I'd been through, and when out and about (with makeup on), even at this point, I looked perfectly fine. Still, two of my docs believed I was teetering on the edge as well and might not make it more than a year or two since a body can only fight so much. Regardless, I was committed to living a healthy life right up until the end, whenever that came.

Back to the headache. As was typical, I was lying in bed and talking to my friend on speakerphone while we were doing all the exercises needed to make the headache disappear when my friend said she saw a couple of strange somethings penetrating my skull. In my mind's eye, I could see it too. Eventually we both saw more than one, and I would start the description and she would finish it. I would mention one location and she'd mention another I had also seen. There was no doubt we were both aware of the same phenomenon. They were shaped like railroad spikes but with short roots. They were deeply embedded. I know it sounds bizarre, but we spent a long time working diligently to remove them from my head. If anybody had walked in, they would have thought I was nuts. Before you concur, read just a little further.

The process we used dealt with focused imagery, and as progress was made, we both recognized it at the same time. One of those invaders was so stubborn to remove that it made me feel nauseous as it fought desperately to hold on while the angels, my friend, and I worked to remove it. Yes, we enlisted angels to help, and a couple of hours later, the three objects were gone.

I know you're all questioning this, so just bear with me a little longer.

We did some healing work around the remaining indentations, and I rested. Neither of us had any idea what might result, if anything, but we both knew it was critical get those things out of my head! My headache had disappeared, but throughout our discussion, it became apparent that I had fallen victim to some sort of psychic attack many years prior. I'm not the only person who now believes such things are possible.

There are many articles from and about Deborah King, *New York Times* best-selling health and wellness author, speaker, and attorney regarding psychic attacks and dark, negative energy on the internet. I found several and couldn't settle on which one to quote here, so I'm just giving her as a potential source for confirmation. Such a phenomenon does occur and it's not as rare as it seems.

Although I do routinely clear myself of dark and negative energy and have done so for many years, this attack was more direct, more severe, and must have slipped in well before I became more sophisticated about clearing. In fact, after a meditation on the subject, I was told this began affecting me in early 1999. Ironically, that was when I began feeling weak, and my first bout of leukemia was diagnosed that August.

When I asked for the source of that attack, it all traced back to my early healing years when I learned to keep my mind clear to minimize pain. When one's mind is active, pain intensifies, so I did the opposite as often as I could, especially when I experienced pain. Eventually, my mind stayed quiet, and I could easily live in the present moment, which is the perfect state

Through that time, I developed my clairaudient gifts, and if people want to learn more about that, they can always visit my website or read my other books. Suffice it to say, one can attract both the good and the bad when hearing the "whispers." Divine guidance comes routinely, but occasionally something much darker shows up. I have an idea of when this may have happened, but regardless of how, something has been trying to do me in for eighteen years.

Here is the miraculous part. Within two weeks after my remote headache and psychic healing session with my dear friend (the first for both of us), my energy was improving. I was still getting my weekly or biweekly blood draws, and my CBC numbers kept doing remarkably better. By the third week, they were perfectly normal. That was August 2017. I was stunned but I guess not surprised. Nothing about the world of alternative medicine ever surprises me.

When I saw my oncologist a couple of weeks later and he reviewed the chart of my blood work, his jaw dropped. I didn't give him details, but none of my doctors are ever surprised by my eventual recoveries. I've had perfect blood work ever since.

So, dear readers, never doubt anything that might come your way. We just aren't smart enough to know all the answers that exist in God's magnificent world. We may not understand what is happening, but we don't have to. Sometimes simply *what is*, is more important than how or why it is.

Chapter 8

YOUR BEST FRIEND— THE BODY MIRACLE

When you don't know who to trust regarding your health, there is one source that will always be right—your body—and it will be right 100 percent of the time. That magnificent, God-given machine is your best friend on earth and is the one representation of the Divine you literally carry around with you every minute of the day.

For the most part, we ignore our bodies unless we're gauging its weight, wishing we had thicker hair, or struggling to fit into a pair of jeans. When we look in the mirror, what do we see? Do you define yourself by your attractiveness or your healthy glow? I know, nobody looks for the glow even though most of us understand that real beauty comes from the inside out. It's just inside beauty doesn't count when we're staring at the reflection of a body or face in the mirror that doesn't make us happy.

You're not alone. Join the millions and millions of people, just like you, who believe their bodies are only composed of the physical, which is used to function and present some perception of who we are. That's why we miss or ignore the body's greatest gifts.

Let's try to change that by considering this. When we first came into this world, each of us had only one thing with us—our body. This unique package—this miracle machine—was our first birthday gift, the one given to us by God. It is, without question, the most ingenious mechanism ever devised. To punctuate that point even more strongly, science and medicine still can't figure it out.

Just think about it—if we were living in a much more primitive society, our body would be our only tool for survival. Its instincts would have led us to nourishment and protected us from harm. We would have nurtured it by keeping it clean, grooming it, sheltering it from the elements, and sustaining it with food. We would have treated it with respect.

Instead, we were born at a much more sophisticated time, and yet with all the education and worldliness we've acquired, we're totally ignorant about the most important tool we were given for survival. Yes, even in this modern age—the body is still a survival tool with parts of it so complex, we've still barely tapped into them.

We take our bodies for granted. We push them to the limits, don't feed them properly, rarely give them the rest they need, fill them full of drugs and chemicals to mask their normal reactions, and rarely listen to the signals they share with us every day. The only time we pay attention to our physical selves is when we look into the mirror or when it's acting up. And then, like I said before, our thoughts are calculating or critical; we are either too fat or too thin, we are getting wrinkles, our ears stick out, or there is some other flaw that we wish didn't exist. When we complain about how these bodies of ours are beginning to break down, how they don't operate as well as they did when we were younger—we focus on the negatives, not the positives. Yet, we forget we're partially to blame for whatever condition they're in. Yes, most of us take better care of our cars than we do with the machine in which we live.

For a change, let's consider our body from a different point of view because that instrument will be your most trusted partner in healing since it guides you and reports on the progress you're making. To drive home that point, here is an example of a few of the wondrous functions this body performs every single day.

The body miracle.

Our bodies are so smart for when we begin to reach for something hot—if we barely touch the searing heat—this body jerks our hand or arm back instantly. We don't have to think about it or give ourselves some conscious command; this happens automatically. While walking along a road, if a speeding car swerves too close, our bodies react, again, and we jump out of the way in a split second. This is automatic too. We don't say, "Gee, that car is coming awfully close, I had better get out of the way," since by then we'd be toast. Our bodies' reactions happen instantaneously—without any intellectual thought and without analyzing the situation. Our bodies help us survive.

Our bodies also do a million other things for us in a twenty-four-hour period and routinely do dozens of them all at the same time. We can be walking down the street with a friend, and at the same time, seeing and appreciating the surrounding scenery, hearing the background noise, chewing and tasting the gum in our mouths as well as breathing and swallowing too. It all happens simultaneously while we're also engrossed in conversation. We might also be digesting a late breakfast and fighting off a cold we were exposed to a couple of days before—all at precisely the same time. We don't consciously plan any of that, and we don't think about any of it while it's happening. Even the steps we take are synchronized and spontaneous—all beautifully orchestrated and managed without any conscious or intellectual effort.

It's amazing when we take time to reflect on the extraordinary gifts we were all given at birth. Just the routine stuff is a miracle, but what happens with a minor scrape or cut, for example, our bodies call up their healing properties. Your blood vessels, blood cells, and skin cells all begin working together to stop the bleeding, prevent infection, and heal the wound. Before long, the bleeding completely subsides, and within a day or two, the skin has permanently closed shut. What could have become a scar over time fades into a fine line that eventually disappears. We didn't think about that, it happens all by itself.

Our bodies also provide us with a built-in pharmacy. When all systems are working properly, we have the capability to internally manufacture all the drugs we'd ever need for anything. Our bodies produce adrenaline when we're under extreme stress and need extra energy or strength, antibiotics when we need to fight off infection, and their own morphine to dull pain. Brain chemicals that help us be happy are called dopamine, oxytocin, serotonin, and endorphins. Our bodies routinely produce whatever is required to fight bacteria, viruses, cancers, and other invaders that pop up inside us all the time whether through some genetic quirk or by accident. Our system of healing is continual. More about that amazing immune system in a moment.

Our bodies also hold an enormous reserve of miraculous power we've not begun to tap. Some mystics, shamans, masters in martial arts, and those who demonstrate the paranormal have managed extraordinary feats by tapping into the power of the very same body we were all given. They haven't been provided with any new gifts; they've just learned to access the ones we all have. They bend metal with their minds, levitate objects, walk on burning coals without pain, and break concrete blocks with a bare hand. Others elevate their body temperature, so they're able to swim in freezing cold water with no protective clothing. Still others use their psychic powers and clairvoyant or clairaudient gifts to see the future or communicate with the "other side." When tested to its farthest limits, our bodies are capable of unbelievable things; in fact, their potential is practically limitless. What else would you expect? We were created in God's image.

Knowing all of this is possible and recognizing that locked within our bodies are resources we have not yet begun to access, why should we ever doubt that our bodies have the capability to heal themselves? The body you and I were given is a miracles—our very own miracle. And, if you provide what it requires, listen to it and pay attention to its signals. This body of yours will not let you down; it will be the one that guides you and eventually heals you completely. All you need to do is respond to its simple requests, and it will keep you healthy.

A couple of examples of signals.

One of the more simple, obvious signals your body provides to help lead you to answers or point you to issues that need resolving is pain, which usually indicates swelling, something out of alignment, or a nerve issue, among other things. Coughs can mean something is in our lungs we need to expel, there is an irritation somewhere causing that reaction, or it is just a signal that we need to check further. Fever means our body is try-ing to eliminate an infection.

Unfortunately, in today's world we don't think about these symptoms as being signals to direct us to some other issue. These signals are now annoyances, and even our doctors are trained to stop the signal and eliminate the symptom. For example, we take a pill to eliminate the moderate fever and an antibiotic to stop the infection instead of letting a moderate fever do its job, as people did years ago. There are lots of examples of this, but today we're impatient, we want a quick fix, but when we eliminate symptoms time after time and never get to the root cause of an issue, the end result is a chronic condition or worse.

How your body speaks to you through illness or accidents.

Louise Hay, a noted author, publisher, and voice on alternative healing, wrote a classic book many years ago titled *You Can Heal Your Life*. In this book, she lists the emotional root causes of almost any issue faced from a specific illness to something affecting a particular body part. She is one of a couple of authors who refer to this specific connection.

The emotional factor is a critical link in mind-body-spirit medicine. As you are probably aware, there are three levels in which we heal holistically—the physical, emotional, or mental and spiritual—so, the emotional cannot be ignored. Her book is a terrific one, which I highly recommend for a quick reference. When something happens to your body, she believes, and I concur, your body is trying to signal that it's time for a change or improvement in your life.

Interestingly, realizing what the emotional root cause is doesn't necessarily rid your body of the disease immediately, but making the appropriate adjustment to your belief system or attitude might serve as a prophylactic for further similar issues or might help mitigate the condition over time.

When she lists the potential root causes, she lists multiple ones. Not all will apply, but as you read through the list one will resonate stronger. That one is yours. As important as connecting with one's body is, connecting with the intuition is helpful too. God provided us with both gifts.

Here are a couple of interesting examples. A knee injury, for example, represents pride and ego and could indicate stubbornness, the inability to physically bend a joint, fear, inflexibility, or that the individual will rarely give in. So, can you see how being aware of what is happening to your body can help you grow and improve as a person? She also provides affirmations to help. I rarely used the affirmations she suggests, but some people like them.

A few more interesting examples are an ingrown toenail—worry and guilt about your right to move forward; lower back issues—fear of money or lack of financial support; nausea—fear, or rejecting an idea or experience; and finally, nosebleeds—a need for recognition, feeling unrecognized and unnoticed, or crying for love. As I mentioned before, although multiple issues are listed, not all of them will apply, so it's important to review the list carefully. No thinking is required; the right one will jump out at you. Sometimes just being aware of the cause and recognizing the changes that should occur will help stimulate the healing process.

The connection from emotional health to physical healing.

Here is one example of how an emotional root cause can be tied to helping a person improve physically—a fun example illustrating the practicality of it all.

I used to go to a fantastic nail tech for years and years, whom I'll refer to as Bill. Later into our relationship, he shared with me that he had high cholesterol issues. I said nothing at the time, but when I went home, I pulled out Louise Hay's book,

In Bill's case, Louise's book offered two probable causes for high cholesterol. They were (1) clogging the channels of joy or (2) fear of accepting joy. I also knew Bill well, and he was structured in his life, although he was so personable nobody noticed. He always planned and rarely ventured too far away from the path he had set. Not too far in the future, he and his partner were headed for a weekend away to a new destination.

On my next nail appointment, and before Bill's pending trip, I gently suggested he try something totally different—to become completely spontaneous. Start out the day with no agenda at all, wander the streets, explore stores or sights that felt right at the time. Allow himself to be more impulsive during the entire trip. Wherever they ended up at dinnertime, look for a nearby place that was appealing and pop in for dinner. No plans since this would be a weekend of adventure. I mentioned nothing about maintaining his normal dietary restrictions.

I believed his energy flow was too restricted and didn't allow for surprises and joy to capture him unexpectedly, which is the only way they occur. That process always stimulates healing. I believed this change might help loosen him up and help his arteries become less closed off or narrow so perhaps the cholesterol issue would begin to change as well. Nothing scientific here, believe me. This was just strong feeling I had.

This is how Bill described what happened in writing in a later testimonial: "I had been struggling with high cholesterol and was very resistant to taking prescription medication. When Sandy suggested what I should do, I got goosebumps all over and knew she was right. Much later, I experimented with her recommendation on a weekend trip where I paid no attention to my diet. The following week my cholesterol had dropped from 224 to 206." Can you imagine what his readings might be if he lived his life that way continually—with less firm planning and more spontaneity?

Doing emotional work on the body is never the total answer, but it is part of the puzzle that illustrates how comprehensively the body functions and how interconnected everything truly is—how we feel, our lifestyle habits, and our belief systems, just for starters.

Our bodies give us messages all the time, and through physical accidents that affect certain body parts, we find insight. If we're smart, we learn from them and benefit in the long term. Sometimes the interpretations are tricky to get, but you might be inspired there too. Here are only a handful of common issues and what their probable causes might be. See if any apply to you. Generally, only one will apply. Thank you, Louise Hay.

High blood pressure. Long-standing emotional problem not solved. With this one, whatever issue pops in your head when you read the statement is the issue that needs resolving. That's the way all this works—once you read the issue, something will pop into your head. Pay attention to that information.

High cholesterol—Clogging the channels of joy. Fear of accepting joy.

Osteoarthritis—Feeling unloved. Criticism. Resentment.

Diabetes—Longing for what might have been. A great need to control. Deep sorrow. No sweetness left.

Fatigue—Resistance, boredom. Lack of love for what one does.

The language of feelings.

Feelings emanate internally from our bodies. We judge our feelings about one subject or another by the way our bodies spontaneously respond. When we well up with tears or cry, we're sad or highly emotional about an issue. When we smile or laugh out loud, we're obviously happy or our funny bone has been tickled. Sometimes we generate some animated facial expression that is unexplainable to others—but we know exactly what that face means! All these expressions of feeling are ways our bodies are communicating with us—sometimes for our own benefit and sometimes for the benefit of others. The ones so far are from the neck up.

Other feelings we have seem to stem from a deeper core in our bodies. As we rush though life, we often overlook many of these feeling signals we routinely get because we're either too busy or we're one of those individuals who've developed the bad habit of stuffing and storing emotions. Yes, some folks push aside their true feelings, especially about unpleasant experiences, and bury them in some dark emotional pit they've created. Who knows where these feelings end up, but since those feelings are generally distressing, it's likely an ugly place.

When we decide to stuff and store natural feelings that occur, it makes learning from these valuable bits of body communication impossible. I have many friends high up in the corporate world who are expert at this process—maybe not always stuffing and storing, but clearly compartmentalizing.

When feelings are continually stuffed and stored, it's difficult to get back in touch with them, and we often find ourselves easily triggered much later and overreacting to harmless incidents and don't know why. Therefore, the person who gets the brunt of the later outburst is simply receiving all the stored anger that was never released years prior to a mother, father, other close friend, or boss. Do you see how that works? Such delayed overreactions cause more stress in our lives, and stress weakens our immune systems. Stress always weakens our immunity because it puts a strain on it.

Most of our feelings take place in the center of our bodies. We are all familiar with the term "gut feelings" or "gut instincts." So, let's start there. Not only do the gut and brain have common chemical elements but, if you notice, the configuration of those two regions of the body is also similar. Some Eastern cultures believe that the messages being sent from the lower center of the body (small and large intestines) are even *more* important than the conscious thoughts from the brain. The gut feelings or instincts are more subtle but produce a sort of "knowing." When we "know" that something doesn't feel right, it probably isn't. That's how accurate our bodies are.

Moving up the body to the stomach area, here is another one you might remember. The "gnawing in the pit of your stomach" or sometimes growling is also very common. Typically, either of those means we're hungry, or in other words, our bodies want to be fed.

"A knot in your stomach" is another familiar feeling. That can also be described as an "anxious feeling" or panicky feeling in the pit of the stomach. That generally occurs when you feel rushed for time, if you're not prepared for something that's about to happen, if you've been blindsided by an unexpected question you can't answer. That's the message your body sends when it reminds you that you've been put on the spot and you're not prepared. Nobody ever wants that feeling, so the lesson here is to always be prepared, and with your planning, allow yourself enough time or keep yourself out of potentially blindsiding situations in the future, so you don't have to put your body through that exercise again.

Another is when your chest feels like it's "closing up." This one occurs right in the center of your breastbone and produces an urgent and panicky feeling. This is a different kind of panic from what I just explained—this is a physical panic when your body is telling you that you're physically in the wrong place. It doesn't want you there. I know this feeling well.

My body happens to be sensitive to some toxic smells like bug spray, oil-based paint, and some perfumes—obviously because of one ingredient or another. The worst for me may be cigarette smoke—even the faint toxicity that exists when I walk into a perfectly ventilated casino, the car of a smoker, or a hotel room that isn't nonsmoking. It's subtle but my body panics, my chest closes, I involuntarily stop breathing (can't control that one), and my body rushes me to the nearest exit. It is an urgent and immediate response that I can't do a thing about except to respond. My body is totally in control on issues like these.

"Heartache" is another beauty. That one I'm sure we've all felt after a loss, separation, or breakup of an important relationship—sometimes a serious misunderstanding between friends. This feeling is aptly named since your heart literally aches. The key is merely acknowledging the feeling by taking some action to relieve the pain. The action doesn't have to resolve the situation, although sometimes it does. Other times it's just to help you release the stress caused by the event. The feeling will then subside. Here are a few examples of what often helps. It's always trial and error until the feeling disappears.

Crying is sometimes helpful. If not, contacting the other person with humility to try to right the wrong—it may not work, but often your body feels relief for acting on the matter. Another is just calling someone you love or miss just to hear their voice on voicemail. You could also write a letter that you never send to release your own feelings of sorrow and sadness. Or just talking to a neutral friend is sometimes helpful—to release the pressure.

In the case of grief or loss, I found some married couples who lost their mates switched to sleeping on their spouse's side of the bed. The goal is to give your body relief from the feeling, and in doing so, you'll be acting precisely like you are supposed to under the circumstances. When your body feels at peace, you've done the right thing whether the result isn't what you hoped for at that moment or not.

There is also "anxious anticipation," a feeling of anticipation that typically foretells of something just around the corner that generally ends up being surprisingly good or even wonderful. It's a little stress and a little excitement all wrapped up into one. Like stage fright. When this feeling hits, don't let it paralyze you. That is a *good* signal and should encourage you to forge ahead. Stare fear in the face and take the next step. Whatever the result, this action is most always beneficial to your growth.

Finally, there's a feeling everyone gets when something important has finally been accomplished and you know it's perfect—whether it's the proposal, poem, or painting. You know when it's finished, and you sit back with a smile. At the end, maybe you get goosebumps, chills, or well up with tears. For me it was when I was spot-on with an ad campaign that had been created—right then, I'd get chills and I knew it would create miracles, and it always did. Whatever it is for you, when that special feeling hits, there is no question—you know it's perfection.

Conversely, when things aren't right, and you know the person in front of you is lying or something else is really off, what signals does your body give? Do your eyes immediately dart to another person in the room for confirmation or support? Do you freeze for a split second almost stunned in silence? Do you furrow your brow? Do you look down or look away? To each of us the reaction can be quite different, but we all have involuntary reactions to unpleasantries in our lives too. If it happens often enough, we'll eventually get the message and maybe make choices to limit similar exposure to that source in the future.

Watch little children. No mistake what they're feeling.

Our bodies have always talked to us, and as children we were instantaneously responsive. That was the joy of childhood. We had no filters and expressed emotions freely, never getting into trouble if our actions didn't hurt anyone else. We were just living life with authenticity.

As toddlers, expressing feelings naturally was adorable. We'd jump up and down when we saw something that made us happy. We'd push things away we didn't like. We were spontaneous, real, and alive. As we grew into adulthood, our enthusiasm for life was tampered down by our parents, corporate protocols, or political disciplines that encouraged us to suppress our feelings—sometimes to mask them totally for such a long period of time that we lost touch with them altogether. We began to let our brains begin to take over without remembering that our bodies are a balancing act between which brain we use and when—the top one or the bottom one, the gut.

There is something special about internally recapturing the joys of childhood. That feeling allows us to see the humor in things others become angry about, allows us to love unconditionally, and allows us to lighten our spirit enough to release stress.

Your body warning you about your health.

Throughout my adult life, I'd been receiving signals from my body about my health, but like most of you, I ignored them. When my eyes would begin to feel heavy at 6:30 at night because I was so exhausted, I'd just drink some caffeine or smoke cigarettes and continue to forge ahead. When I was anxious and overstressed, I sedated myself with alcohol to calm down and relax; instead of releasing the stress, I masked it. I pushed and pushed and pushed for years ignoring anything that had to do with my body and me. I always put myself last. And, finally, my body gave me a major wake-up call. Those attacks of excruciating pain in various joints in the middle of the night eventually morphed into rheumatoid arthritis. Because I wasn't listening to the whispers, my body had to yell.

If you experience continual feelings of discomfort in your body, it could be a pattern to which you need to pay attention. The goal is to get rid of discomfort when it happens. Your body is trying to help. It wants to feel perfect and feel at peace continually. In that state, healing, regeneration, and growth are in the optimum environment. In trying to reach or perhaps maintain that goal, your body communicates with you so it can share exactly what it needs and when it needs it. This process is the opposite of masking the feelings artificially or being driven by habit, which is the way most of us operate.

The first time I can remember consciously noticing my body speaking to me was the experience I shared earlier with the methotrexate and my rheumatologist. When he suggested that therapy, my body froze momentarily; I couldn't say yes or no for a minute, I just looked at him. My second reaction was to pull back, to pull away. I didn't think at that moment—I felt. That is when I told him I needed some time, left, and began my journey. My body was right. It told me to pause before reacting and take some time. That advice was right for me!

Don't ignore your feelings, they are there to provide guidance. Feelings are the language of the soul.

Your body's action signals.

Some of the most fascinating signals are the ones that aren't feelings at all but are instead actions. Involuntary actions you don't even notice happening until they're over. Pay attention to your life from now on and notice when you do something automatically that reveals how helpful your body can really be.

On more than one occasion, my body walked me into a place I never would have considered going. You know, "the devil made me do it" compulsion. Once, I was *drawn* into a health food store. It was one of those old, cluttered, and dusty ones, not the kind of environment in which I would ever enjoy browsing, but I automatically walked in. That is where I met a wonderful contact in the back room who became a valuable teacher who helped me explore several mysteries in the world of alternatives—many I still use today.

Unrelated to healing, here's another situation that involved my former husband, Steve. One afternoon, Steve was headed home down the freeway and was in sort of a zone while driving. I always kidded him about being a Pisces and being prone to zones anyway, but during this instance, his car was being pulled off at an earlier exit from our normal turnoff to head home. This exit was at Indian School Road. He caught himself as the car began turning onto the off-ramp, and he whipped the car back to the left, nearly colliding with another car, so he could head the direction he considered to be the right one on the freeway. Before he got to our normal exit, his car phone rang (at the time there were car phones, not cell phones), and it was a client who had papers ready for him to sign. Guess where the client's office was? Yep, it was east, just off the Indian School Road exit.

On another occasion, the signal came in the form of a specific body movement. I guess you could also call it a *reaction*. You know when your head turns involuntarily and you catch sight of something that's important for some reason? That is precisely what happened to me just not long ago when leaving my house for a meeting. I'd finished getting dressed and was walking through the dining room to head for the back door when my head turned, for no apparent reason, and I noticed a folder on a nearby chair that was important for that meeting. I'd have clearly forgotten it without the nudge. So, I smiled, grabbed the folder, said *thank you*, and left for my meeting. I'm eternally grateful for the guidance I receive over and over throughout the day, but unfortunately, most people are too preoccupied to notice.

One more to share. A good friend and past business associate of mine had just flown in from Denver that day and stopped by my house as we had arranged. We were going to run down the street and grab a quick bite to eat before calling a client of ours in Australia, who had a fifteen-hour time difference. The call needed to happen at 7:00 p.m. MST in time to catch him at the start of his business day. While we were standing in the kitchen, my friend's arm rose slightly and she unconsciously looked at her watch and said, "Oh, it's five forty-five, we still have plenty of time for dinner and to call at seven. Let's go." I wasn't wearing a watch, but since my friend was, I wasn't concerned.

We returned home from dinner in plenty of time and made the call promptly at 7:00 p.m., but we found we were an hour too late—our client had already left for a meeting. My friend had forgotten to reset her watch from Denver time when she arrived in Phoenix, so her watch was an hour behind. We should have made the call at 6:00 p.m. PM Denver time. Her body tried to remind her to check her watch and notice the time difference. A nice reminder, but neither of us connected the dots.

Fascinating how our bodies remind us to do things that might make lives flow easier and simpler. Hopefully now readers will begin to pay more attention.

Spontaneous thought and our bodies.

Since the body is our best friend in all things healing, we must realize all good friendships rely on effective communication. You might be curious about one particular method of communication that needs no interpretation since it is surprisingly direct.

Spontaneous thought is a the most obvious way our bodies facilitate communication. Now whether that original thought emanates from the subconscious mind or superconscious mind (the state of wisdom and intuition)—which some might interpret as a Divine source—doesn't matter because that source can be whatever you want it to be. It is there, however, and cannot be denied. We've all heard it. It is that quiet, little voice that comes from somewhere inside us to guide us routinely. That's the voice that sometimes says *"Speak up"* or *"That's a bad idea."* Yes, we've all heard something like that.

I heard that voice pop into my head as I was walking down the aisle at my first marriage—a formal wedding, no less—on my father's arm. About halfway down the aisle I heard, *"Sandy, what are you doing?"* Boy, I pushed that thought away quickly since I really didn't want to hear that one at this point. The quick end to that story is that after two years and no children, we called it quits. Yep, that relationship should have been a date, but we were both so very young. No harm, no foul.

Since these are not conscious thoughts, we have nothing to say about the timing, and it's much easier to receive such information if one's mind is uncluttered, so I encourage people to begin the day with a quiet mind and then remember how residing there feels, so they can continue to maintain a blank mind throughout the day. When the mind is not tasked with worrying, ruminating over issues, or singing songs in our heads, thoughts that come spontaneously are easier to recognize. Those are what I call the whispers, and they are generally wise, loving, and always very helpful.

When random thoughts pop into my mind, they are usually important. Sometimes they're answers to questions I wondered about out loud earlier. For example: I had been concerned about a great gift to get someone I knew. I sort of asked the question with a strong thought and then forgot it. Within a short period of time, although it sometimes happens instantly, the answer or idea comes.

There are other common examples about how random thoughts guide us. I could be in the shower and there's a flash in my mind to remind me that I still have clothes in the dryer. A clear mind can help you receive those wonderfully practical messages and the ones that will help guide you to through your day and to better health.

The body and dreams.

We're still not finished; there are dreams too. Dreams are part of our built-in inner guidance systems. Dreams were never critical in my healing messaging back then, but they are to many others I've known. However, there was a brief period when I was going to a Jungian counselor who asked me to write down the dreams I remembered for her later interpretation. So, I kept a pad and pencil by my bed to record them quickly before I forgot. That experience with that counselor were incredible.

A quote from Carl Jung, the Swiss psychiatrist and founder of analytical psychology, has a wonderful quote about dreams: "Who looks outside, dreams; who looks inside, awakes." He also believed dreams are not meaningless and they often carry their own unique way of expressing themselves.

I am not an expert on dreams and never really used them in my healing work, but I do realize how powerful they are in communicating with us. One particularly vivid dream was interpreted by that Jungian counselor I visited for a few months. I had dreamed that a woman I knew had her feet sticking out from under the dust ruffle on my bed. As I pulled her out (by her feet), she was stone cold dead. I wasn't shocked, it was simply what it was.

After sharing that dream with the counselor, she asked what this woman represented in my life, and I told her that she was the quintessential socialite. Well, it appears this dream was giving me notice that the socialite part of my life was over. That was 2007 or 2008, and it ended up being precisely the case. I had been very high profile in that arena, but it wasn't my total life, just a part. My involvement lasted decades, but now due to the limits from my illnesses and resulting financial status, my life was changing.

I was grateful for the heads-up since it is very easy for people to try to reach back to revive what may have been part of one's life in the past. I didn't try so that saved me a lot of wasted energy over something that was never critical to my life.

So, dreams can warn us, prophesize, bring advice on improving our lives, relationships, and health as well as connect us with loved ones who have passed. Dreams are wonderful, and if you're drawn to that subject, there is a whole world there that awaits!

Kinesiology and other methods of communication.

Finally, one of the most powerful ways our bodies communicate to us and others is with kinesiology, a method of muscle testing many chiropractors use to ask our bodies for information. For me, kinesiology was one of the first and most dramatic illustrations of body talk. With that method, my chiropractor knows which vertebra has which issue and which organs need help. No mistakes with that method—and no wasted time.

Our bodies can also facilitate communication with a pendulum. Some might consider that New Age mysticism, but dangling a string with a ring dangling from it over a pregnant woman's stomach to determine the sex of the baby is an old wives' tale for gender prediction that dates back centuries. In fact, any object that hangs from a string or metal chain, when suspended from a stationary position, will automatically swing back and forth or in a circular motion. Those movements can be interpreted differently by each person to provide yes and no answers to basic questions regarding health, healing, or other personal growth issues. This requires a little training so one's mind is always clear, there is no investment in the answer, and you clearly understand for you what each movement means (they can be different from one person to another). This can just be a shortcut to quick answers on frequency or strength of supplementation and to prequalify methodology for which one's in doubt. Its application is limitless except for lottery numbers, picking horses, and other gambling reasons. Tried it—doesn't work for those. ☺

Christiane Northrup, MD, the nationally recognized holistic expert in women's health, believes that listening to your body is one of the five immediate steps you can take to heal yourself. "That means tuning-in and taking care of yourself. Start by resting when you're tired. And eating when you're hungry. And saying no when you've reached your limits. The more you honor these internal messages, the more inner guidance will come your way. As your powers of intuition develop, you'll soon know what your body wants and needs. It's uncanny—but 100% reliable." (57)

Chapter 9
YOUR IMMUNE POWER

The immune system controls our body's healing on a physical level. It can be the key to recovering from many diseases and conditions that range from fibromyalgia, chronic fatigue, and infections to cancer. The more we learn about this incredible, internal system—the more we can take control and make better choices to help our bodies heal.

The immune system works on behalf of each of us 24/7, but it can also work against each person or not be helpful at all, such as in the case of autoimmune diseases. Autoimmune diseases occur when the immune response—instead of being directed to an invader—becomes misdirected and focuses its aggression against the body's own tissues or organs. In other words, the immune system goes haywire and attacks the body. When that occurs, the immune system can negatively impact nerves, joints, endocrine glands, connective tissue, skin, or muscles, causing a variety of different conditions.

There are more than one hundred known autoimmune diseases with some of the most common being type 1 diabetes, RA, psoriasis, multiple sclerosis, lupus, Addison's disease, inflammatory bowel disease, myasthenia gravis, Graves' disease, Hashimoto's thyroiditis, celiac disease, pernicious anemia, Guillain-Barré syndrome, as well as endometriosis, fibromyalgia, Lyme disease (chronic), myocarditis, restless leg syndrome, rheumatic fever, scleroderma, vitiligo, and vasculitis. There are many others.

Not everyone who has an autoimmune condition has ever been told their condition comes from an immune system that isn't operating correctly, which is unfortunate because then patients might otherwise begin to learn more about and pay more attention to their immunity. I think that is a failing in a system that needs to help patients become savvier about preventive care.

There are also diseases called immune deficiency diseases, which occur because the immune system becomes deficient or weakened. The most notorious are HIV-AIDS, chronic fatigue syndrome, and Epstein-Barr, which are virus-based diseases or conditions that have been allowed to progress. An immune system that is temporarily weak may also set us up for a host of other virus-based conditions such as the notorious hantavirus, bird flu, mononucleosis, West Nile virus, SARS, and our latest viral outbreak, COVID-19. Less traumatic but equally stubborn can be the common cold, respiratory virus, influenza, and herpes simplex and herpes zoster. The list for viruses might also include infectious rabies, measles, warts, and mumps.

Although there are more than two hundred primary immunodeficiency disorders, when our immune systems are weak, we become vulnerable to a host of issues including bacteria that can be air or food borne, cancers, and conditions caused by parasites, fungi, or microorganisms. Still, we can be protected from all of these with a healthy immune system that destroys those culprits before they can destroy us. None of the conditions I have mentioned stand a chance if our internal defense mechanisms are in top form.

Now, are you beginning to realize how important a healthy, functioning immune system is? Sadly, physicians do a poor job of educating their patients about the immune system in general. If they did, we'd all be paying more attention and asking what we could do to help ourselves.

I've been an example of doing something most conventional medical providers would say is impossible—that being to bring my immune system back to working order after autoimmune or immune deficiency issues—and I've done so naturally. If one's immune system has ever been normal even though suffering from one or more autoimmune diseases or immunodeficiency diseases, it's possible for the natural function to return to that incredible system. It can be done once or multiple times. Since our cells have memories, if we give them what they need without taxing our bodies in the process, we can regain good health if we've ever had it before. Again, if you ask your doctor, I'm sure he or she will disagree—which is why the title of my first book was *Get Well: Even When You've Been Told You Can't*. I've taught myself all the disciplines that need to fall into place to keep my immune system functioning normally. It might not be a common occurrence—it might be very challenging to accomplish—but it is possible. I am a living example of that.

Conventional medicine has had little or no success offering cures for autoimmune or immune deficiency diseases other than to shut down a person's immune system, making it more vulnerable to everything else it could be fighting. Seems like a lousy option to me.

Science through the pharmaceutical industry has spent billions of dollars over the years focusing on killing the disease with drugs and not helping patients naturally strengthen their body's own immune systems. When we do the latter, the former rarely occurs.

The same with cancer. We've spent billions on research to cure cancer when cancer takes so many different forms. If we spent one tenth of that on educating the public about how to keep their immune systems in top shape, that miraculous system would be killing the malignant cells before they ever took hold. A perfect segue to the next section.

Are you sure cancer isn't different?

No, cancer has a direct relationship to the immune system too. One of the jobs of the immune system is to scan cells to eliminate anything that does not belong in the body. As I mentioned before, this surveillance system weeds out malignant cells too. So, if cancer appears, it's not because we caught it from another person or from something floating in the air, it's because there has been a significant failure in our internal surveillance system.

According to Andrew Weil, MD, in his early book, *Spontaneous Healing*, "Cancer only attacks us when our immune system becomes suppressed or depressed and our routine 'surveillance mechanism' breaks down. If there is cancer in your body, even in its earliest stages, it represents a significant failure in your healing system." (58)

"If someone has cancer, conventional treatment can do very little except offer surgery, radiation or chemotherapy." Dr. Andrew Weil continued, "Only the first procedure makes any sense at all, for removing the cancerous growth, if possible. The second two are crude treatments that will be obsolete before long. If someone chooses radiation or chemotherapy, there will be damage to their immune system. The question in selecting treatments like these is whether the damage done to the cancer justifies the damage done to the immune system." (59)

If a patient has an early-stage cancer or a chronic form, there is so much time to let the body do a little of the work while making it stronger in the process if you ever decide to endure chemotherapy or radiation therapy. As we all know, choosing chemotherapy and radiation is always the patient's choice, and although your oncologist may state that option as a matter of fact, it's not the doctor's choice.

Again, I'm not advocating that someone with a cancer diagnosis do it my way since a person must do what their body is calling them to do, not what they are being pressured in to. But though many might prefer to delay such radical forms of treatment, they don't because they don't know of any other option that might really work. After a diagnosis, take a breath before making any decision. Do a little research first—perhaps a second opinion from someone in the more natural arena—then decide. If you have the time, it might be worth it. One option is to look for a naturopathic oncologist, who can recommend different options but would also be available to work with your oncologist (many do) to keep your body as healthy as possible while you venture out into the conventional route of care.

Diving headfirst into the unknown may have been something I was willing to do, but I am certainly not recommending that option for anyone else.

Cancer remains a dreaded disease that puts fear into the hearts of nearly everyone receiving the diagnosis. Unfortunately, please remember that fear is one of the emotions that also weakens the immune system, which becomes a problem itself. Attitudes that generate a feeling of powerlessness can compromise the immune system by robbing a person's body of the energy it needs to sustain good health. So, the quicker a person decides not to let the fear of any disease overtake them and instead commit that they're going to overtake the disease, they begin to regain the energy or power needed to strengthen the system designed to fight this condition, as well as others.

The power of our immune systems is extraordinary. If you want more detail about how to keep it healthy and want to know specifics, this next section is a good place to begin.

What weakens and strengthens the immune system?

At some point in my journeys, I decided to look back and see if there was any pattern to what I did to help my immune system heal. There was. This is a proprietary list that I created in early 2000 after reflecting on my many journeys. This didn't come from any physician or health care provider, either conventional or allopathic. No doctor has ever educated me about my immune system or offered suggestions that directly relate, although they have certainly told patients to drink less, get more sleep, or exercise more—perhaps even made dietary suggestions like cutting back on salt or eating more fiber to help with cholesterol. Still, the recommendations they make are never tied back to why this is important for one's immune health. Those suggestions are also always disease specific, based on a current diagnosis—they are almost never general preventive suggestions.

The only person who ever came close to educating me at all was the amazing nutritionist back in the '80s who did tell me that all drugs interfere with the functioning of a healthy immune system. So, again, this is how I kept and keep my immune system functioning properly, and I'm delighted to share it with you.

The elements have been broken into three separate segments: those of a physical nature (BODY), those of an emotional or mental nature (MIND), and those of a spiritual nature (SPIRIT). Yes, that's mind-body-spirit medicine or, in other words, holistic healing. Our bodies are so complex that all elements are intertwined, and each affects the other. It's that comprehensiveness that amazes me and why I like to call it my miracle machine.

Although the original list comes without annotations, I added a few here so readers could grasp the point being made more clearly. Hopefully you'll find those comments helpful.

WHAT WEAKENS AND STRENGTHS
THE IMMUNE SYSTEM

Weakens		Strengthens
BODY	Physical Stress such as environmental pollution, loud noise and chemicals	Calm, peaceful atmosphere
	Excess Candida Albicans	

Candida Albicans is a fungus that lives in the body and is found in the intestines, skin, and mouth, primarily. It can also show up in other parts of the body like the vagina, typically known then as a yeast infection. The question isn't if a person has Candida but how much Candida a person has. When the condition becomes systemic, it can interfere with organs and negatively affect one's immune systems.

Drugs—illegal, prescription caffeine, tobacco, alcohol	No drugs

All drugs impact our immune systems, so if a person is trying to heal from a chronic or very serious condition (not routine or smaller issues), stopping all drugs is helpful, so the immune system can begin to heal and self-regulate. You will know when and if you can ease back to any of those listed, such as alcohol, caffeine, and a prescription drug here and there.

Chemicals in foods—dyes preservatives, aspartame	Healthy, fresh, or frozen food

Read the labels. If you can't pronounce most of the ingredients, it's smart to pass. These chemicals will not be healing to the body, they will do just the opposite.

Food allergies or sensitivities

You can identify sensitivities by severely limiting your diet to the most basic proteins and green vegetables for a week and then slowly adding back one of the most common culprits at a time: wheat, gluten, corn, dairy, caffeine, sulfites and nitrites or other food preservatives, aspartame, MSG, food colorings, sugar alcohols (zero-calorie alternatives to sugar), and eggs, for example. Since that takes a while, some prefer the shortcut, which is identifying something you eat frequently and is a dominant part of your diet. Keep track of everything you eat and drink for two weeks, then look back. The foods that dominate your life will show up. Eliminate that one food for a week or so and see if symptoms improve. If that's not the issue, try another, and so on.

Lack of sleep	Good quality sleep
Vitamin and mineral deficiencies	Replenish/enhance body nutrients (vitamins, minerals, enzymes)

Most humans are deficient in a vitamin or mineral here and there. Testing is beneficial, by a naturopath, osteopath, or holistic medical provider. Supplement what is lacking so you can regain a normal baseline. Continue the supplementation because you're deficient, remember? One day's dose doesn't shore up an empty reservoir, which you draw from constantly.

MIND	Fear-based emotions	Love-based emotions
	(i.e., fear, anger, resentment, guilt, hatred, impatience, greed, jealousy, worry, etc.)	(i.e., love, forgiveness, compassion, gratitude, kindness, humor, support, trust, etc.)
	Attitude—negative	Attitude—positive
	Stress—emotional	Release daily emotional stress

The more a person focuses on things that irritate or stress them, the more likely those issues are to stick with you. Try to find outlets for normal stress like exercise, walking or running, healthy sex, long baths, and meditation.

Release stored, negative emotions

These are more difficult to release because people who "stuff and store" emotions rarely recognize they do so. They end up with a stockpile of stored negative emotions with which they haven't dealt or released. That can result in disease and pain. To learn how to release them, there are a variety of alternative providers with solutions, articles on the internet, and although I used to do in-person workshops, perhaps I'll do something one day online.

Mental therapies—affirmations, visualization

Self-Love

SPIRIT   Hopelessness   Faith and Trust

I'll say more about this in later chapters, but one thing is for sure, your spiritual body might have the most serious impact to your health, and immediately so. People can subconsciously "will" themselves to die and not be aware of the cause when serious symptoms do erupt. Feeling hopeless about your life, an illness, or giving up on the process of living can be fatal. Details coming up.

Simply remember to avoid everything on the left side of this list and embrace everything on the right is the ideal path to take. When attempting to recover from long-standing, chronic, or very serious issues, you'll want to follow this closely. There will be more about the specific minerals and vitamins that help strengthen immunity in a later chapter.

There are several other tips that will also help strengthen your immune function, and some involve common sense. Remember to laugh, pray, welcome love, and try to live a balanced life. Take deep breaths and spend time with close friends.

Keeping good bacteria in your intestinal tract is smart too—probiotics or prebiotics are generally needed supplements. Some social cultures are smart enough to introduce acidophilus in their foods routinely, like dill pickles (kosher), sauerkraut (German), and miso soup (Japanese).

The more you know, the healthier you'll become.

Chapter 10

THE VIRUS MYSTIQUE
AND ANSWERS

The reason the COVID-19 pandemic didn't frighten me much is that I understood how viruses behave and what a person needs to do to protect themselves against them. My education about viruses has been ongoing over the last forty years because with an unpredictable immune system, I've always been vulnerable. The moment I felt the slightest discomfort in my body like the beginning of a bug, I'd start paying attention to what my body needed and would respond accordingly. Over time, I managed to assemble a first aid kit of antiviral remedies as well as remedies for other symptoms I was having and take whatever I needed when it was appropriate. I felt totally empowered throughout the time everyone else faced panic.

In terms of the vaccine, I'm reluctant to get into the "vaccine" debate other than to state that these shots are still experimental whether they've been approved or not because the pharmaceutical companies are still gathering data and continuing to learn. Additionally, the fact that pharmaceutical companies keep issuing booster after booster within such short periods of time and without any human testing is concerning to me. It's like an amateur shooter at a gun range scattering bullets everywhere hoping to land a couple in the bullseye. Without the adequate preparation necessary to approach that arena, it is painful to watch. In the case of these vaccines, it might also be painful to experience.

NBC News reported in August 2022 that "the vaccine boosters, issued around Labor Day 2022 would be the first COVID shots distributed with only mice trial data and no results from human trials. Although some compare updating with boosters being similar to how vaccines for the flu are modified each year, yet other doctors disagree stating that influenza shots are based on decades of experiences with strain changes whereas the flu vaccines behaved generally the same way. With these, it's the first iteration of the COVID vaccines and the mRNA technology has only been used since late 2020. No question experts disagree on the 'huge assumptions' the agency is making." (60)

The public seems to be responding accordingly since not everyone is rushing to receive all the new boosters being introduced unless they are mandated by some entity, and then many do so reluctantly whether approved by the FDA or not.

I've had a bias against of the FDA and certainly pharmaceuticals for decades.

Part of my resistance to clutch in desperation to whatever the FDA or pharmaceutical companies throw out there is that I've had little trust in the process of testing, approving, and overall efficacy of pharmaceutical drugs since the 1980s. I feel I should further explain that, so readers have full disclosure and are free to discount the parts of the text with which they strongly disagree.

Here's my beef regarding the FDA's drug approval process. The FDA has approved a multitude of drugs over the years, and some have still been pulled off the shelves years later because the side effects ended up being much more severe than were initially reported.

Initial test results aren't always conclusive as long-term side effects often surface. I bring up this drug as an example because we are all familiar with the name, but there are still dozens of others I could mention but won't.

"VIOXX (Rofecoxib), which was approved in 1999 as an anti-inflammatory medicine used to treat arthritis, was a product of Merck. When it was pulled off the shelves it already been prescribed to over twenty million people who as a result suffered profound side effects including stomach ulcers and bleeding, strokes, and heart attacks. A study by the government, asserted that VIOXX was linked to over 27,000 heart attacks and cardiac deaths during its time on the market. It was finally pulled in 2004." (61)

This time, with rushed approval, I had even less confidence in the mRNA technology, which prior to this time had been completely untried in human beings for a coronavirus. Although mRNA vaccines had been tested against rabies in 2017 in Germany, in 2019 two vaccines against influenza and one against cytomegalovirus were also tested, and there was interim data from the mRNA vaccine against Zika, which didn't make me comfortable.

Just because a drug was tested doesn't mean a thing without hearing the results. The results from the rabies and flu mRNA vaccines "were somewhat modest, leading to more cautious expectations about the translation of preclinical success to the clinic." The team noted that in both trials, immunogenicity was "more modest in humans than was expected based on animal models … and the side effects were not trivial." (62)

From those results pharmaceutical companies rushed into human trials, which were exactly what the launch of the mRNA technology was. Even worse, the mRNA trials happened on the world stage, and throughout these companies have continually pushed the boundaries of age to access them, whether there was a risk warranted or not—especially to younger groups.

From the article quoted in chapter 4, which appeared in *Natural News*, titled "'Science' no longer trustworthy: BMJ op-ed suggests all health research should be considered fraudulent until proven otherwise," here is another quote from that same article. Ben Mol, professor of obstetrics and gynecology at Monash Health, talks about his forty-year concern about research fraud noting that "at least 20 percent of the time, reviewers and editors of journals are wrong in assuming that the results of a given trial are honestly reported." He continued, "In many cases, trials that are reported to journals never actually happened in the first place. Someone just made the whole thing up to push a new pharmaceutical drug or medical device, for instance." (55)

So, with that bias, you may ask if I was vaccinated myself.

I guess that's a logical question at this point, but with my bias against pharmaceuticals for more than thirty years, I don't think anyone would be surprised that I passed and have not been vaccinated. Throughout the push and, in some cases, mandates to become vaccinated, I passed. Even though I fell into the high-risk group being immunocompromised and being over seventy-five years of age, I wasn't gripped by fear, and even though I ignored the vaccine chatter, I did reluctantly but dutifully comply with each of the other mandates and requirements.

I wore a mask when it was required, but only then. I was out and about from day one, except for the brief stay-at-home phase. I ate in restaurants that remained open and never wore a mask outside or while alone. I behaved myself but thought most of the hysteria was overblown.

Avoiding the fear helped keep my immune system from becoming more vulnerable from the paranoia that seemed to grip everyone else. I maintained my sense of humor and continued with my normal healthy lifestyle.

What I did was one thing, and if people were to ask me what I thought, I'd advise folks (and did do so) to wait. Today, I am not recommending readers vaccinate or get boosters or not. By this time, it's a moot point since everybody has made their own decisions.

Still, regardless of your vaccine status, if you are someone who'd like to become more empowered with your health, this book is designed to provide tools to do so. For readers who have been vaccinated, boosted, and are facing buyer's remorse, I encourage you to research a number of the medical mavericks mentioned earlier who have begun to explore remedies that might be effective to counter some of the unintended consequences of these shots. It's worth research, regardless.

You're probably also curious if I ever contracted COVID-19!

Not for nearly three years. I sailed through the worst of it, and although I had to be tested a couple of times to attend events, the tests always came back negative. Then in late fall of 2022, COVID finally caught up to me. No real warning on this one, in which case I could have jumped into my antiviral routine—this one just came on, fever and all, in a few short hours.

I was facing some extra stress in my life, and the holidays were approaching—always red flags for me—and the week prior a pap smear tested positive for E.Coli and strep even though the symptoms I was experiencing were practically nil. Then, within a few days of that diagnosis, when my body was fighting those, I became overchilled at a lengthy outdoor event and was somehow exposed to the coronavirus. Even the best of us become vulnerable when the stars align against us.

Once I received the test results, I attacked the COVID issue with off-label therapeutics, a couple in-home mega-Meyers IV cocktails, which included vitamins C, B-12, and B complex as well as zinc, magnesium, and glutathione. I drank lots of fluids, used an over-the-counter expectorant to keep the cough loose and productive, replaced electrolytes with Pedialyte and used a handheld nebulizer, as I'll describe later, to neutralize respiratory issues. Even though taste was an issue, I made myself eat a little each day. It took more than a couple of weeks to fully recover.

Regarding the GYN issue, since I don't react well to antibiotics, I used boric acid vaginal suppositories to change my pH balance so my body would become more alkaline and could deal with whatever infection still existed from that source. After I'd improved from the COVID, I added a couple of my antiviral remedies—a few of which work for bacteria as well.

Readers will find my complete list of antiviral remedies next, which I hope will provide a good starting point to become more empowered to live day to day without fear.

I know you're all curious, so here are the natural antiviral remedies I use.

The key to warding off the cold, viruses, and other bugs is to catch them very, very early through preventive techniques of when the first slightest signal appears. Most people wait too long. So, let's begin with prevention first. To keep my body functioning perfectly, I take several different supplements, but specifically to bolster my body's immune fighting power, I take these.

Vitamin C—Vitamin C is a necessity for every adult. It is smart to take daily, not just when you're feeling poorly. This is my go-to vitamin since I used it for healing from my leukemia (in therapeutic doses both IV and oral), and because of that, I take much higher levels daily than most people would. However, most normal adults typically require 2,000 mg a day. 1,000 mg in the morning and 1,000 with dinner. Über-healthy folks can get away with 1,000 a day. The reason that dose is so high is because stress reduces vitamin C levels because we all now live in a stress-induced society.

I prefer a buffered C powder, but buffered capsules are good too. If you've never taken vitamin C with any regularity, jumping to 2,000 mg a day might be too difficult for your system. The side effect is loose stool, so if that occurs, taper off until your body adjusts. You might start with 1,000 a day and work up. 500 mg in the morning and 500 mg in the evening, then increase to 1,000 twice a day after a week or so.

As I've stated before, most in conventional medicine have no idea how lifestyle, stress levels, or anything else depletes the levels of vitamins and minerals in our bodies. That's evident by the minimum daily requirement the medical community recommends. In the case of vitamin C, it is merely 90 mg a day, which is woefully deficient for any real benefit. So, if you take that dose, it's a waste of your money.

The above illustration is why I'd never ask an MD, unless he or she is a holistic provider, anything about dosage or even the subject of supplementation. Always check with a naturopath, holistic MD, chiropractor with nutritional training, or another alternative provider. You could also simply read articles regarding natural healing from the internet. Friends with lots of experience might also be helpful since we are not playing with lethal drugs here.

I obviously take much higher doses because of my vulnerability and the fact my body is used to more and now seems to require it. If I cut back, I catch colds more readily and often become constipated—also not good.

Zinc—This one I also take daily, but it can be confusing since there are lots of zinc formulations: zinc picolinate, zinc citrate, zinc glycinate, and zinc chelate. Some work better for one person than another, which is why trained professionals (from naturopaths, holistic MDs, osteopaths, and even a few chiropractors) might suggest one over another for you. However, zinc glycinate is what I currently take and seems to be what is most popular with docs I know these days. These come in 20 mg capsules, but that is way too low of a daily dose. I take from 120–150 mg daily (two to three times daily), but people should not take less than 50 mg, or again, it would likely just be a waste of money.

Vitamin D3—Much of the population is vitamin D deficient. One reason is that we've slathered on sunscreen for so many years and blocked the healthy rays from the sun. So, there are two options to get your daily dose of D3—either sit in the sun (without sunscreen) for twenty minutes a day or take a supplement. I frankly think supplements are easiest, or you could do both. Obviously, don't sit in the sun during the heat of the day—mornings before 10:00 a.m. are best in states like Arizona, Nevada, Hawaii, New Mexico, and even in Southern California. I happen to take 5,000 mg in gelcap form. I take two 5,000 mg gelcaps a day, but many people do well with only 5,000 mg total per day. There is no need to take more than 10,000 a day, ever, without the possibility of toxic side effects, which will easily occur when one reaches the 20,000–50,000 mg doses. More is not always better.

Magnesium—Also good and any deficiency of this mineral may contribute to ADHD. Magnesium deficiency can cause anxiety or trouble sleeping, so if you suffer from either of those, magnesium might be helpful. Magnesium is also important for the absorption of vitamin D and is helpful for people with occasional constipation.

Vitamin B Complex—This vitamin helps maintain a healthy immune system too, and the B12 and B6 within are particularly effective for preventing shingles. This vitamin becomes depleted with a stressful lifestyle or if you generate stress in your own life, which is very easy to for the readers who are worriers. For the shingles virus, B vitamins are particularly prophylactic.

If you feel like you're catching a bug.

At the first sign of any cold or flu symptoms, these are the remedies I have on hand, and I take them immediately since I know they will progress.

Even allergy symptoms can cause fluid buildup in nasal passages, and in those fluids, over time, viruses or bacteria can begin to breed. I deal with allergy symptoms quickly so they don't grow into something more.

Postnasal drip is often the sign of a sinus infection, a scratchy throat is typically a rhinovirus developing, and lymph glands that feel a little tender and swollen are another sign of viral invaders. At the first sign of a cold, I am never very concerned—I simply select the best remedy for the symptom and then remember to get enough sleep, stop alcohol intake or anything else that could weaken me over the next day or two, and eat well, and whatever it is disappears. No need to take all these remedies at once unless the virus progresses over a couple of days and seems to be getting worse.

ZICAM Nasal Swabs will kill the nasal virus on contact and are a great natural remedy that can be found at your local drugstore. Zinc (the ZI in ZICAM) is miraculous in that regard, so sometimes with early allergy symptoms (that can eventually lead to a viral infection), I use these zinc remedies as a preventive. You can obviously see the benefit of killing nasal viruses immediately. Take as directed. Another option is the nasal spray or the lozenges. I like the swabs myself.

ZICAM Rapid melts are also good. They are also at your pharmacy and you can select your favorite flavor. The zinc will kill germs in the throat caused from postnasal drip, or the start of an aching or scratchy throat. This will stop the virus before it migrates to the chest.

Sambucus Elderberry Syrup. Take as directed, and this comes in a bottle. It's yummy tasting, so simply put 1 tsp in 2 oz of water. This is a natural antiviral and is very effective at the first sign of a virus (which can also simply be the common cold). You'll buy this at a health food store, Sprouts, Whole Foods, or another natural market.

North American Herb & Spice Oil of Oregano. I am being specific as to the brand because not all oil of oregano is created equal. This one is very high quality. Also, if you are certain that you are coming down with something, take two drops in 2 oz of water and chug it. If you don't, it will burn your tongue and taste dreadful if used without water. Although this oil doesn't dissolve in water, water serves as a good carrier to make it possible to toss this mixture down your throat like a shot of very bad whisky. Twice a day. One in the morning and once at night.

There is a second form of this oil by North American Herb & Spice called H2Orega, micellized oil of oregano, which is a water-soluble type and dissolves more quickly in water. Some prefer this one. Either are fine.

North American Brand Oregamax capsules. Depending upon the severity of your symptoms, you can take up to three capsules with each meal, three times a day. Both the oil and the capsules kill everything! Within two or three days, you should feel perfect!

Zand brand zinc lozenges. You can buy these at Sprouts, Whole Foods, or other health food stores. They are for symptomatic relief only. You can take them one after the other since they are the zinc topicals that kill viruses on contact and make it possible to swallow, even with a bad sore throat. However, you need to make sure you read the packaging carefully since it is easy to pick up the orange flavored one by mistake, which is only vitamin C. They also have elderberry, which is a general antiviral but very weak. What you want for bad sore throats is the zinc, which is the lemon flavored.

Vitamin C. Mentioning this again, since if you catch a doozy of a cold that comes on quickly, you can take half your daily dose of vitamin C, which might be 500 mg or 1,000 mg, three times a day or up to every three hours. Discontinue if your stool becomes loose and let your body recover for a few hours.

Supplement for one more virus.

I am only listing in this section supplements with which I have had direct experience. Other sources you might find helpful are some of the more famous integrative, physician-owned websites, although I must caution you that most all have branded products that feature combined ingredients and become very confusing. A person could also go bankrupt taking everything that is being offered to help us maintain a healthier lifestyle. These are all simple solutions and cost efficient.

Cold sores are the presence of the herpes simplex virus. Taking lysine has always proved helpful to me. There are now lysine creams, which I have never tried. Also, once I began taking this harmless supplement when an outbreak occurred, a therapeutic dose, they just disappeared after a few days. You might check online for suggested dosages or talk to a knowledgeable health food provider or alternative practitioner.

Homeopathic remedies that are terrific for other issues too.

My first go-to remedies are generally homeopathic remedies since they can be carried in your pocket or purse anywhere, are totally harmless, and work instantly. Homeopathic remedies work much like old-fashioned vaccines in that they are based on two unconventional theories. "Like cures like"—the notion that a disease can be cured by a substance that produces similar symptoms in healthy people. Or like old vaccines, which introduced the similar condition into a person's body to stimulate the immune system to produce antibodies to fight the issue. Homeopathic remedies work so quickly it's amazing.

The second theory of homeopathy is "law of minimum dose"—the notion that the lower the dose of the medication, the greater its effectiveness. In fact, many homeopathic products are so diluted that no molecules of the original substance remain. Hard to explain unless you understand the power of energy. I use them all the time, and when my son died, I wasn't sure I could make it through the funeral composed, so I called my homeopath, and she told me to pick up a remedy at Sprouts on the way. I did what she suggested, took one dose, and in an hour took another. I was composed for the entire day. I wasn't dopey or drugged, I merely regained my equilibrium so I could function normally.

The brand I prefer is BOIRON for homeopathic remedies. They are available online or at Sprouts or other health food stores. However, it's important to understand how to take them since they come in a little cylinder-shaped container with a cap on one end. Inside you'll find tiny, round sugar pellets we used to have in our doctor kits as kids. With the cap pointed down, twist the cap so five pellets drop into the cap. You will want no more, no less. If more than five fall into the cap—pull the cap off gently and slowly tap one or two pellets back into the container. Do not touch a pellet or it will become contaminated. Do not touch the rim of the cap to anything or it will also become contaminated. Pull the cap off slowly, so the pellets stay in the cap and then toss the pellets under your tongue and let them dissolve.

These remedies come in two strengths—30 c or 6 c. I always buy 30 c, which is stronger and for more general use.

For postnasal drip. BOIRON Brand. Hydrastis Canadensis: 30c

For spasmatic cough. BOIRON Brand. Pertussinum: 30c

For allergic or viral runny nose. BOIRON Brand. Allium cepa: 30c

Flu-like symptoms: body aches, headache, fever, chills, fatigue. Homeopathic remedy that comes in its own box. It is called Oscillococcinum. It is not a BOIRON product but is the best on the market for the flu. Take as directed—but when it says "dissolve entire contents of one tube in the mouth every six hours," they mean under the tongue. It is not to float around a person's mouth. Holding them under your tongue allows them to absorb into your bloodstream more quickly.

Note that flu symptoms are often much different from cold or simple virus symptoms. With flu a person can run a fever, feel achy all over, and feel tired. Sometimes there is nausea too. Colds, sinus infections, and such mainly present with pressure in the sinuses, runny or stuffed noses, a scratchy throat, and sometimes a cough. So, Oscillococcinum is a flu remedy.

There are so many other remedies that are remarkable for everything from indigestion, nausea, and bloating to allergies, sinus issues, and depression and grief. You can even find them also for food poisoning or bruises and even the rapid healing of bone breaks. I love homeopathy for day-to-day issues.

All the remedies I mention here can be ordered online through sources online like Vita Cost, which has good prices, quick delivery in the US, and free delivery for any order over fifty dollars, health food stores, natural groceries like Sprouts and Whole Foods and health food stores. I never buy vitamins at normal grocery or drug stores. I find the brands they carry aren't always the highest quality, and their buyers don't do the due diligence needed to ensure higher-quality products.

However, drug stores are fine for the over-the-counter remedies I mentioned above and for some homeopathic remedies you'll find advertised on TV like Highlands Leg Cramps or homeopathic products for urinary tract infections and a few others. If you read the labels carefully, they will note they are homeopathic, even if ingested like a typical pill. Homeopathic products aren't as far out there as you may think.

Happy healing!

Chapter 11
MIND-BODY-SPIRIT (HOLISTIC) MEDICINE

Mind-body-spirit medicine isn't very complicated to understand since it's all spelled out in the name. What makes the process complex is how those elements work together to heal us completely by interacting with one another. The good news is that we don't need to understand precisely how it works, we just need to grasp the concept in general. That will all become clearer in this chapter, especially when comparing differences between scientific-based, conventional medicine and mind-body-spirit medicine.

We need to begin with a vocabulary lesson since most people interchange words that aren't interchangeable and become confused by myriad terms.

Let's begin with conventional medicine.

First, let's get a few other terms I've referred to out of the way so you understand exactly what they mean. Throughout this book I will describe the scientific medical model as conventional medicine and sometimes allopathic medicine. They are one and the same. Scientific medical practitioners use the initials MD after their name or in some case have indications for their specialty of care such as OB-GYN. Both conventional and allopathic are correct references.

Traditional medicine is not a term to describe this form of care since conventional medicine is less than three hundred years old. Traditional medicine describes methods of care that have lasted a very long time and have been used for centuries or millennia to treat patients such as many forms of care in the alternative world. In other words, used through tradition.

When conventional medical providers want to appear open and flexible to the alternative worlds, they may use the terms holistic to describe their practices. Candidly, these end up being more integrative in nature than holistic. MDs use the term integrative as well and, in this form, will occasionally blend or suggest methods like massage, acupuncture, chiropractic, and nutrition into their treatment plan. The spiritual, mental-emotion and the way these two elements work collectively to heal are rarely considered or even understood in conventional medicine.

If given a choice and I had to stick with conventional medical doctors, I'd always choose those who are more integrative or claim to be holistic.

Back to mind-body-spirit terminology.

Holistic healing and mind-body-spirit medicine are one and the same. Both involve the whole of the human body: the physical body, the emotional and mental body, and the spiritual body. They work together to heal on a very profound and intricate level.

Now to the actual terms people use to describe the alternative world. Some use the words natural medicine or naturopathic, some say homeopathic (meaning holistic), and some say holistic. People rarely casually refer to the process as mind-body-spirit medicine. It's just too cumbersome for casual dialogue, although it reads well for marketing purposes. Yet only one of those words describes healing the whole body, and it's this one.

Holistic means the whole, emphasizing the comprehensive nature of healing on all three levels instead of focusing solely on the physical body. So, when this word is used in the context of healing, it refers to considering the impact of how a person thinks, feels, responds, and behaves, and specific lifestyle habits they demonstrate in their care. Each of those very different functions impacts a person's physical health.

Homeopathic means something totally different. Homeopathic is a method of treatment that is one of dozens that exist in the world of alternative medicine. Homeopathic is the adjective used to describe homeopathy, which is the modality itself. Homeopath is the person who treats; therefore, the homeopath is the provider.

The practice of homeopathy is totally unique to any other modality that exists among alternative options, as I mentioned earlier. This system of treatment based on using highly diluted remedies made from natural substances to trigger the body's own immune response mechanism into action. It is basically harmless because the medicines or remedies it employs are very diluted but effective for a range of problems. Homeopathy can work on the physical body, the emotional body, and the spiritual body, as well—usually with simple tiny round pellets that dissolve quickly under the tongue. A variety of practitioners can practice homeopathy—those who are licensed and certified are referred to as homeopaths.

Natural medicine is a descriptor of any form of alternative care that exclusively uses nature and God's gifts as its source for treatment such as hands-on therapies, herbs, massage, acupuncture, exercise, and nutritional counseling and could include homeopathic remedies and other therapies such as hydrotherapy (colonics) and so on. A provider does not have to be a naturopathic physician to provide natural medical therapies.

Naturopathy is a separate category of alternative care, like homeopathy. In the United States, twenty-six jurisdictions license and regulate naturopathic doctors. Providers complete a four-year course at an accredited naturopathic school. This practice primarily focuses on reforming the patient's diet and lifestyle, adding supplementation of vitamins and minerals if needed, and often referring patients to a wide range of other alternative modalities as mentioned above, sometimes performing one or two of them personally. Naturopaths are the providers of naturopathy.

The term we'll be using most often in this section is holistic since that word describes the mind-body-spirit process of delivering health care.

How are holistic healing and conventional medicine different?

The fastest way to gain a complete understanding of what holistic healing is to compare it to what it is not. So, in the following you will find the categories that differentiate these methods—the comparison should become crystal clear.

Length of an office visit is a good place to begin. With holistic healing, you'll find the provider will spend as much time as it takes with a patient—listening—with a half hour to hour-long appointments not unusual. The appointment time is longer so holistic providers rarely are as highly compensated. Conventional medical providers spend much less time with patients, on average thirteen to twenty-four minutes. (63)

Focus of practice is also a fascinating subject. Holistic providers tend to consider what person has the disease rather than what disease the person has. I'm paraphrasing a quote from Hippocrates, who had the same philosophy. On the other hand, conventional medicine tends to focus on the condition or illness and spends less time getting to know the patient. One practice is patient focused and the other is disease focused. Scientific medicine attacks the disease or condition whereas the holistic provider develops ways to nurture and support the body so the body, often through its immune system, can do the work itself. A totally different training.

Healing time will be an important category for people expecting instant gratification. With holistic care, healing is cumulative and progressive and generally takes longer. This method is also more comprehensive. Conventional medicine, on the other hand, appeals to individuals seeking a quick fix and who are content with Band-Aid-type cures for their symptoms. In this arena, physicians rarely get to the heart of the condition to remove it permanently. Since conventional medical cures are typically symptomatic, they allow for chronic conditions to remain. Years later the patient is still sick. That method of care is good for the doctor but not great for the patient.

Comparison of therapies is another way to measure the difference between holistic providers in the alternative world and the scientific medical approach. Scientific conventional medicine works with lethal tools, drugs that run the risk of side effects—some minor and some very serious—surgery, which is invasive and requires prolong healing, and radiation, which like surgery not only damages the immune system, but while killing the cancer cells it also kills the healthy cells nearby. The risk of medical mistakes is nonexistent in alternative medicine since the treatments they use nurture the body, not destroy it.

Personal responsibility is where a huge difference exists. Conventional physicians let patients off the hook as they gladly assume the power position in the relationship. The patient runs to the doctor to heal them or cure them—abdicating complete responsibility themselves. Conversely, in holistic care, the patient and physician work in collaboration to do what they can to help the patient's body work most efficiently and effectively. The goal is for the body to become fit enough to fight the disease or condition. The patient does not turn over all power to the physician and instead they work as a team. A totally different treatment model. The holistic physician listens and listens, which is the only way they gain the insight to know which path to recommend. Holistic healing is patient-directed versus physician-directed care.

The gatekeeper for care is another significant distinction. In conventional medicine, the gatekeeper is always the primary care physician—be it general physician or internist. That person controls care and makes referrals if warranted. In the holistic healing process, it's quite different. The patients themselves are the gatekeepers and the holistic providers aren't expected to provide all the answers or even be the key source of referrals to other modalities of care. These providers rarely expect to be exclusive. A naturopath, a holistic MD, and a holistic DO (doctor of osteopathy) can all be primary providers, but some patients go exclusively to homeopaths, Ayurvedic doctors, or those practicing traditional Chinese medicine, among others, as their sole providers. I have had a holistic MD, naturopath, chiropractor, masseuse, hydrotherapist (for colonics), as well as oncologist and others in my Rolodex at the same time. It really depends on the individual patient.

A cure or symptomatic relief also is a distinction in how the provider is comfortable treating. With holistic healing, chronic isn't a word that's widely accepted since providers look for the root cause of conditions and try to help the patient find the core solution, which sometimes involves multiple levels of focus. Very often this process is patient led and intuitive, other times the physician guides the process. Regardless, the patient is free to explore emotional and spiritual methodologies to help solve the problem, not mask the issue with symptomatic relief. Healing is generally lasting since it almost always involves permanent lifestyle change and healing on multiple levels.

Conventional medicine cures the presenting symptoms first and generally stops there, with the exception of when surgery is recommended, and then most solutions are lasting. However, in the case of conditions they refer to as "chronic," which would be all autoimmune or immune deficiency conditions, physicians may stop there or try different pharmaceuticals to remediate the symptoms. If ineffective, they often change prescriptions. Although conventional medical doctors do, holistic physicians rarely accept that some conditions are incurable.

Interestingly, conventional medical providers also use the term remission when referring to cancer not showing up any longer in tests. I believe that is harmful since that word sets up a nagging belief in the patient's subconscious that may be buried but is always there. Such a hanging threat makes the patient more a victim than a victor. Comprehensive healing makes that possibility of any such reoccurrence much less likely, unless the patient's own behavior in the future sets up a possible new onset (much like I did with the leukemia).

More about taking responsibility.

As mentioned in the earlier section, it often takes more than one provider to deal with the complexities of the human body and how the mind, body, and spirit all play a role.

Hippocrates, the father of modern medicine, who was born in 460 BC and died around 377 BC, was credited with freeing medicine from superstition and advanced the idea of preventive medicine. Prevention was first mentioned in *Regimen and Regimen in Acute Diseases*, one of Hippocrates's books, stressing that diet and the patient's way of living could influence his or her health. Today, everyone, including physicians, tends to ignore the details of diet and lifestyle in healing. Yet, holistic providers do and it's in that arena where the patient's personal responsibility enters the picture.

If any of us are honest in looking at the shape our bodies are in today, it wouldn't be a stretch to acknowledge that we may have done some damage to ourselves in the early years. The overworking, the overeating, the overwhelming stress, the drinking, and smoking might also have been factors. For some, it was even drug use in the '60s or yo-yo programs of weight loss that continued throughout their lives. Or the massive amounts of radiation, chemotherapy, and prescription drugs we took or are still taking. Most importantly, not learning how to release stored emotions over the years after stuffing and storing them habitually might also have been a damaging habit. Those abuses chipped away at the magnificent machine we were given, little by little, until we're now left with a weakened version that's beginning to give out. Any wonder?

I could compare such neglect to never changing the oil in your car. When that happens, you end up with sludge and eventually engine breakdown. In the extreme, trying to run your car without oil would really cause disaster. After the horrible screeching from the metal parts slamming into each other, the engine will lock up and stop running, but not before severe damage has been done. Your body is no different.

So maybe you are someone in trouble or are feeling the effects you assume automatically come with age. They do not. If you can admit that the choices you made in the past—and might still be making today—could have contributed to the weakening of your body, you will have just taken the first step toward getting well. If you can acknowledge the power you had to weaken your body, you must also acknowledge the possibility that you have the power to strengthen it too.

Accepting personal responsibility is the first step to taking control of your healing.

Total healing is always cumulative and progressive.

As an example, in my case, I was led to a variety of different solutions for one issue I faced with an autoimmune disease. This process would apply to any autoimmune disease. The process involved bringing my immune system back to normal. It was a complicated process and I happened to discover all those solutions by accident. The potential solutions came randomly as well, and how to keep myself functioning normally and building strength throughout sort of rolled itself out too. Your healing doesn't have to be that mysterious. I'm offering a road map.

The first part of my healing taught me the most. I learned that even though I had a great nutritionist initially, some people wouldn't start there at all. Regardless of where you begin, that source will not and should not be the only source. In my case, that wonderful nutritionist helped me improve about 40 percent, and I was smart enough to continue with what she taught me. I didn't leave her and look for someone who would help me 100 percent. Things don't work that way when a person heals holistically. I was 40 percent better and that was great, but onward and upward.

As I found additional providers in completely different arenas of care, some worked for me, and some didn't. The ones that didn't, I quit seeing. The ones who helped I used for as long as they were helping me make inroads. When I learned all that I needed from that source, I added another. I didn't burn bridges and often I'd return to an old resource for a refresher. But, throughout that journey, the cumulative process of my healing continued.

The next situation brought me about 10 percent improvement. Supplements I was encouraged to add, again coincidentally, helped me another 10 percent. I kept doing all the good things, and now I was 60 percent improved. See how that works? When I started finding emotional, mental, and even spiritual answers—like learning to live in the moment, which totally released stress, and things that used to make me angry now made me laugh. Some I found on my own and some wisdom I gained from others. There is something positive about being open to being led and rising above the panic, anger, worry, and fear that comes with facing illness.

Answers will present themselves in many different forms. With each experience your body will judge its value. Some providers will offer advice about what you should do with your lifestyle or nutritional choices; still others will provide direct remedies. Some will provide spiritual resources and emotional tools. Others may introduce a new alternative method you'd never been exposed to before. I find I'm brought answers when the timing is right. Odds are you'll receive something you need on your journey from every experience you have.

Long story short, after three years, I was totally well from autoimmune issues that had plagued me for at least twenty years and maybe more. Knowing what I did and how that works allows me to stay that way, and if I slip, I remember what to do to recover.

It is always a matter of a little improvement here and there. There is no timeline since as long as you are improving, even a tiny bit, you're headed in the right direction. The thing to remember is don't quit the regimen you have established. Too many people, the minute they start improving, quit what they are doing. That's when they begin to go backward—bad idea. Don't stop what's working.

When you reach 100 percent, don't throw up your hands and say to yourself, *OK, I'm fine now.* You are only fine because you have found a regimen that works for you. Pull that away and your body will backslide.

Most of these are supplements, not cures, they are supplementing a system that needs them. So, because of routine stress and other issues that deplete our nutrients, supplements need to be continually replaced in your system. Again, it's why you check the oil in your car and have it changed every six thousand miles.

It's not my fault; it's in the genes.

Some people try to excuse their illness based on a family history of one condition or another. Genetics are no excuse for becoming ill. Yes, I can explain that.

Although some people are very lucky and come from a strong gene pool, most of us have multiple chronic or life-threatening ailments somewhere in our family tree. These are potential problems we've inherited from one distant relative or another that might include heart disease, cancers, arthritis, and sometimes even more exotic strains lying in wait in our bodies. Yes, it's not easy dodging the lousy-gene bullet, but it is possible.

If a person has a predisposition to a condition, it does not guarantee they'll contract it, especially if their natural defenses are in good working order. For example, we all have malignant cells floating around within our bodies, but we don't all get cancer. As you remember, one of the jobs of our immune system is to scan cells to recognize and eliminate the bad ones that don't belong there; it routinely weeds out the malignant cells too. We have developed this defense over the course of our evolution, and it works—unless we have weakened our immune systems in one way or another.

In my own case, there was a strong genetic case for my eventual rheumatoid arthritis, which I wasn't aware of until I was in the middle of my healing journey. You see, I'm adopted and didn't meet my biological mother until later in life. It was then revealed to me that on my maternal side, there was an uncle and aunt both severely crippled with rheumatoid arthritis, a female cousin currently suffering with it, and my biological mother has osteoarthritis. Later in life, my half sister now has RA as well. Yet, I have been able to regain my health and live pain free and drug free by keeping my immune system strong enough to keep this weakness from surfacing in my body. Leukemia is also in the family lineage with an uncle who died from it and a cousin currently struggling with the same disease. Yet, my blood work is normal.

Genetic weaknesses can be overcome if we are aware of those conditions and don't exacerbate that predisposition through our own behavior. Even after such a diagnosis, the progression of that condition isn't assumed to be a fait accompli. At the risk of oversimplifying, if we have a propensity for diabetes, we'd eliminate refined sugar, eat a low-glycemic diet, watch our weight, and make sure we get plenty of exercise. If we're prone to heart disease, we watch our diet and cholesterol levels, monitor our weight, and quit smoking—or we wouldn't start some of those in the beginning. Learning how to rid our lives of stress and not generate more stress is also beneficial for everything. Basic education, common sense, and a desire to preserve our bodies is what is needed to maintain good health.

Even if illness does strike, there are steps we can take to help ourselves recover. We have the ultimate control over our health since that control comes from the choices we make every single day. Being aware of our family history is part of the education, but it doesn't sentence us to a life of illness or suffering.

Healing on the emotional level.

Let me share one of my stories that will illustrate how our mental/emotional state plays a role in the physical body's health. That fact became most evident when I quickly healed from my leukemia the first time.

I was doing all I knew to do on the physical level and was successful—well, almost. My white count had dropped to normal after eighteen months, but my lymph count was more stubborn. My energy level wasn't perfect either. Even though I could have pushed my oncologist to drop the leukemia diagnosis since my white count had returned to normal, I knew full well that the lymph count still needed work, and that was the other key marker in the type of leukemia I had. I could have said *make this lymphocytosis* and he would have likely complied, but that wasn't being honest. My LGL leukemia was not yet history.

So, I ran to Louise Hay's book, *You Can Heal Your Life*, to look for the root cause of the leukemia issue, since I still hadn't pursued the emotional element of my healing. There were two core reasons that applied to me—the first explained how my subconscious led me to this physical decline in the first place, which I'll explain in the section of this chapter dealing with how spirituality works in healing. The second for me was lack of joy. Hmm.

Now, all I had to do was remember what joy felt like and begin to recapture that feeling. Well, I couldn't remember what it felt like or even when I truly had joy in my life. I decided to look at old photos to try to identify when I felt truly joyful. So many times I've been happy, I had been excited, I had been and was optimistic and positive, and I was even peaceful and content, but none of these were true joy. In fact, the feeling of joy completely eluded me.

Then my first grandchild was born, and the moment I saw Charlie Cowen in his father's arms—as Jon walked out of the delivery room— something happened to me. His sweet little face looked exactly like his father's did when he was born. For an instant, I was dumbstruck, but simultaneously, something swept over me that I didn't recognize. It was an instantaneous and overwhelming feeling of bliss or something that came from the inside out. It radiated throughout my body in one gigantic burst of emotion. It also gave me a series of continual, gentle soft chills that came in waves. I truly can't describe the feeling—sort of a warmth, I guess—but I knew in that instant I was feeling something extraordinary. It was pure joy.

There was something about recognizing my son, Jon, in Charlie that made me open my heart unconditionally to love that flowed through me from some Divine place straight through to my first grandchild. It was like a power jolt. That jolt of love and bliss were extraordinarily healing. I guess I could feel that but shoved the awareness aside merely delighted to bask in the glow of it all. Within six weeks, my lymph count dropped dramatically, and at the end, I was completely well.

Of course, I must acknowledge that throughout those six weeks, I'd call Jon and Jodie to ask if I could get a Charlie-fix and maybe just watch him while they went somewhere, even the store! Ha. They were kind and would drop him off quite often, and you'd find me sitting there, holding him on the sofa and doing what I said I'd do. I just watched him with my heart wide open, and I was always flooded with joy. Those experiences were constant reminders to me what true joy felt like, and soon I was able to continue that feeling as I opened my heart to other parts of my life: my friendships, a glorious sunset, the magnificent nature all around me, and in daily experiences I had taken for granted.

Ever since, I've privately called Charlie my Joy Boy. Since then, I have been blessed with two other beautiful and very special grandchildren who have magnified that joy enormously. Just a tiny dose of Charlie, Jack, or Lucy—especially since my son's passing in 2018—is all I need in my life to make it complete and totally joyful!

I've been in bliss for nearly twenty-three years since Charlie turns that age in the spring of 2023. Jack is now twenty-one, and Lucy will be seventeen when this book is finally published.

Healing on the spiritual level—and how the reverse is also possible.

I'm leading with something shocking only to illustrate the power of our spiritual selves in the healing process as well as its ability to do extraordinary damage. The spiritual element in our healing can either cure us or kill us. I know that woke a few readers up, and I don't mean to scare anyone, just make us aware. Guess I'd better explain.

The flip side of helping us heal is how our bodies also make it possible for us to subconsciously will ourselves into a death spiral, even when in reflection we don't remember the exact trigger. This is how that phenomenon works—at least in layman's terms.

I am not talking about the nocebo effect by which it is possible to inflict psychosomatic physical damage to a person through their belief system. Example: a person is involved in a clinical study, and that person believes that something harmless (like a placebo sugar pill) can do harm to them instead. In one case a patient took twenty-six placebo sugar pills they imagined were the actual depressants from the study to kill themselves. They had a serious reaction—their blood pressure dropped seriously low, but they survived. That would be a consciously induced situation that could lead to serious harm.

I'm also not talking about suicide or any conscious effort for a person to facilitate their death by not taking medication or something similar.

What I am referring to is not proven by science, but it is a fact of life that I have experienced myself and have witnessed in others. You have also, I'll bet, but don't recognize what you have observed. It's always triggered the same way. A profoundly shocking or devastating experience occurs in one's life that causes a momentary desire to stop existing or wishing their life would end at such a deep soul level that it becomes imprinted into the subconscious as a command, and the body then delivers on that request.

Before you slam this book closed and with certainty and think I'm nuts, bear with me. If you will refer to my Immune System Chart, you will see under spirituality that faith and hope strengthen our immunity (power of life) and hopelessness weakens it. Well, hopelessness, lack of faith, and giving up, at a deep level, weaken it for sure but can also do more than that.

Let me give you one example that happened to a friend of mine, since she shared the total experience with me from the "other side" years later. I had also witnessed her life up close and could see what was happening, although I wasn't sure the reason, but the illness and departure were too quick for coincidence.

I had a strikingly beautiful friend who, along with her husband, had a moderately open marriage. They adored each other but since he had married her when she was merely eighteen, I think he felt she may still need to spread her wings. He never encouraged this behavior but also wasn't jealous and looked the other way occasionally when he could have spoken up. There may have been another reason since this gave him an excuse to take a vacation here and there from his wedding vows himself.

Long story short, the couple also had two sons. One was divorced and still living and the other had passed a few years prior. The son who had died was his mother's favorite. When the adult son passed, it was tough for my friend to take, but she soldiered through. Not long after, she also found out that her husband was fooling around with the remaining son's former wife. This was much too close to home and painful since there was interaction. I believe the combined pain was too much for her to bear, and within a few months, this extraordinarily gorgeous woman at seventy-two developed bone cancer and was dead within the year. In her later message to me, she had planted that wish deep into her subconscious when trying to manage the simultaneous pain but wasn't aware on a conscious level of what she had done.

This truly isn't that uncommon since most of you know of married couples who were so extraordinarily close in their decades-long, beautiful marriages that when one passes the other isn't that far behind. Everyone says the remaining spouse died from a broken heart, but they truly died from the grief and loss they couldn't bear to live with. Eventually the body delivers with a heart attack, rapidly advancing cancer, stroke, or something similar and gives them exactly what they asked for in their very brief but soulful command.

The good news is that this can be reversed, if we become aware of it. My own story illustrates that.

When I tracked the emotional root cause of my leukemia, the trigger for the onset of the disease was brutally killing inspiration or profoundly falling into the "what's the use?" state of being. This is how I developed the leukemia in the first place.

When I thought about it, I was able to identify exactly the time when I subconsciously gave up. I had just experienced a series of days with my husband that left me emotionally exhausted and spiritually bereft. This was a reoccurring event, since I was married to an emotionally abusive man at the time, but since he'd stopped drinking ten years prior, the emotional abuse was occurring much less frequently. I still was reminded of his anger issues, from which he still couldn't recover once a year when he couldn't help himself. He had failed to receive the emotional counseling he needed to truly heal and remained a "dry drunk." I had acquiesced to my life, and I seemed to be able to manage this event once a year.

Your question is likely, what? You're a smart woman, Sandy, and you're all about empowerment. How could you stay? Well, the rest of the year was fun, and my son and husband had an ideal relationship. At the time, since I worked so much and my husband was a great helper, I thought breaking up the family would hurt my relationship with my son. It's always complicated, you know.

This annual event was particularly devastating to me since it's always a matter of the content of the messaging that left me full of pain and numb. The one salvation was always the existence of my son, Jon, my only child, and someone I adored. But at that time, Jon, too, seemed to emotionally abandon me. He was getting married and was captivated by his wife's family, which pulled him away from us more than usual. I felt as though I was losing Jon to another family, but whether that was real or imagined, it didn't matter. Jon and my husband were my only real family since all my other immediate family was gone. Both situations appearing roughly at the same time was too much.

I can remember saying to myself in a split second, as I was distraught and dead serious, *"I can't take this anymore—I don't want to be here."*

Those words came from deep within my core. The grief was so real and both emotional attacks hit simultaneously, which was just too much for me to handle. Obviously, the message landed right smack in the middle of my subconscious, which heard it and acted. That was February 1999. Not long after that incident, my body responded and gave me exactly what I had asked for.

By April, I was so tired I could barely function. Month by month I got weaker and felt worse. By August, I went in for a checkup, and in September, I had the leukemia diagnosis. It was that simple: I said it, my body heard me and then delivered exactly what I'd asked for. You see, we're always responsible. I can give you case study after case study illustrating the same phenomenon. I guess what kept this from killing me was my relentless ability to fight.

The lesson here is if our bodies are that powerful in a destructive way, imagine how powerful they can be in helping us heal.

The positive side of spiritual healing.

Finding a spiritual connection that can accelerate your body's ability to recover or keep you healthy isn't a matter of turning the channel to the right frequency. It often involves a journey in which your body will always act as the facilitator. It seems it just takes us there when we need it most. Being open helps.

We may be drawn to certain books or articles, certain groups of people or religious organizations, or other sources of tapping into the spiritual world. Some spiritual healing encounters evolve with habits and behaviors like embracing alone time or learning to be still after we first wake up to feel how our bodies are responding each morning. I happen to do a little physical inventory, which isn't anything deliberate, but rather involves feeling my body from the inside out to become aware of what might not feel normal. I don't always act on the feeling; I just become aware, and being aware is always a positive thing.

What is ideal is when we can begin to shift from staying in our heads to opening and feeling from the heart as we navigate the day. It's a matter of dropping the intellectual control and trusting more. For some, it's being willing to be led. Believe it or not, our minds often sabotage our efforts to make good choices. We should trust our intuition much more so than what we think. Intuition is a part of the spiritual world. Considering that the gut is configured somewhat like the brain with all those twisty parts wadded together to perform the functions both do. Through the years, I've learned to trust the mass in the middle more than the mass at the top.

The spiritual part of healing is also evident in the providers we choose. As we learn to drop judgments, we continue to grow in a spiritual sense, and we are tested to see how much faith we have. That is particularly evident when we visit alternative providers who might not meet the expectations we held surrounding conventional medical doctors. That was certainly the case with me.

None of the sources who helped me had expensive offices, fancy cars, great-looking eyeglasses, haircuts, or whatever (yes, I noticed those things in the old days). I could tell they didn't have a lot of money and it didn't matter in the long run because most had such special gifts that I couldn't help but trust them implicitly. Throughout my journeys I became less critical of others, myself, and the timing of my healing progress. I began to accept more and judge less. Both of those are spiritual qualities, you know.

It was easy to sense the healing gifts each of these alternative providers were given. They weren't overtly spiritual, not religious or behaving in ways that would have appeared stereotypical to most of us. They just had gifts that were hard to explain—a love, a gentleness, and a healing quality that over time began to reveal itself naturally.

I became more grateful and reached out to a power much greater than I to share that gratitude. Living in gratitude is also a spiritual quality.

As I felt more spiritually connected, I'd ask for guidance routinely. I felt that connectedness as I would lie on an acupuncture table, wait for my Reiki practitioner to finish working on me, or experience the healing effects of essential oils. One couldn't help feeling more bound to the Divine than when I was experiencing an Ayurvedic meal designed just for me, sipping a remarkable Chinese herbal tea, or simply taking time to quiet my mind to relieve stress. Everything in the alternative world always linked me closer to love and healing. Perhaps that's why it all works so well.

I learned to relax, go with the flow, and try to control less. In the process I put fear aside and began to trust more. As one notices the eventual improvement, albeit slowly sometimes, it's easy to accept the timeline—any timeline. If it was moving in the right direction, I was thrilled. With healing, time is never the enemy since plateaus level out when other elements in the healing process need to adjust. I never tried to figure out why my body might need a little more time at one stage or another to do its internal work. I really had no idea; it wasn't up to me to judge.

Most importantly I had faith, eternal faith that answers would come. Not hope that maybe it would happen, but solid faith that knew it would.

Can religious practices become part of this journey too?

Those who are deeply religious can easily reflect on the role religion has always played in helping them in one way or another live longer and choose smarter paths in their lives. The teachings of Mormons, Seventh-day Adventists, and Orthodox Jews all include precautions regarding diet, alcohol, hygiene, and other health-related behaviors known to favorably impact morbidity and mortality. God always wanted us healthy.

Prayer plays a huge role in healing too. Interneciary prayer has always been particularly powerful, and its wonderful prayer groups are often called upon to pray for someone at a critical stage. Many miracles have been documented to the power of prayer.

Rituals also trigger emotions that, in turn, often lead to changes in better health by positively impacting the immune and cardiovascular systems. In fact, the psychodynamics of faith can be indistinguishable from the placebo effect.

We can't overlook the laying on of hands or other ritualized activities practiced by healers native to many cultures, or even those in the Western Hemisphere who have been given gifts in that field. Much of that process can be tied to stimulating an endocrine or immune response facilitative of healing.

Meditations and some abstentions such as intermittent fasting may also promote health. Many of those stem from religious or spiritual teachings.

One of the great experts in the field of prayer and spirituality in healing is Larry Dossey, MD, the author of thirteen books, several of which are *New York Times* best sellers, but one of his earliest is the source, not verbatim but paraphrased, for many of the elements I listed above. His book *Healing Words: The Power of Prayer and The Practice of Medicine* is a must read for beginners wishing to explore the new world of alternative methods. Although published by HarperCollins in 1993, this book is one I consider foundational for establishing a solid understanding of the power of connecting with the Divine to help us find our way back to health.

After meeting him years ago, Larry Dossey was kind enough to endorse one of my books.

There is formal research to reaffirm that spiritual practices and spirituality in general are good for both mental health and physical health as affirmed first by the NIH physician-researchers David B. Larson and Susan S. Larson. That team, who found after a twelve-year period of surveying, published in the *American Journal of Psychiatry* and *Archives of General Psychiatry* that participation in religious ceremony, social support, prayer, and relationship with God had a positive benefit in 92 percent of the cases, neutral benefit in 4 percent of the cases, and negative effect in 4 percent of cases. Similar findings for physical health, in research by F. C. Craigie and his colleagues, in a 1990 review of ten years of publication of the *Journal of Family Practice*, 83 percent of the studies showed benefit, 17 percent were neutral, and none showed harm. (64)

The method by which individuals weave the process of spiritual experience into their overall healing varies, but there is no doubt doing so will produce benefits. If healing is needed in someone's spiritual life, it will be beneficial to that person's overall physical, mental, and emotional healing too. For me, the natural progression of my healing—on every health issue I faced—included a strong element of spiritual connectivity and growth. You, too, will find that same connectedness occurring. It just happens during lengthy journeys.

As I mentioned before, some people are already linked solidly to the spiritual, and in such cases, trust and faith will come easily. For others, it will take time and will unfold in a way that will feel comfortable for you, and which you'll be able to accept.

Progress will come when during the quiet time, the silent time, the alone time. When you begin to quiet your mind and learn meditation, you will be able to listen more intently and read your body more readily. Quite often then your Higher Power or Higher Self will also talk to you through spontaneous thought. I like to believe the Holy Spirit has guided me throughout.

As you surrender to your journey and become humble in this process, it will be amazing what develops because of all the intense emotional work, physical adjustments, and reawakening faith. I expanded my creative self, got clear on my purpose, and found peace and contentment I had never felt before in my adult life. Probably the most remarkable results were the intuitive gifts that appeared; those shocked me. That may or may not happen for anyone else.

Through this remarkable journey, you may begin to see and then become overwhelmed with gratitude for a life that does not have to be a struggle at all. All the answers are there. We simply must ask, and they come—sometimes in odd forms—but who are we to judge?

Chapter 12

STEPS FOR ANSWERS TO COMPLICATED ISSUES

This chapter is especially powerful for people facing issues like any autoimmune issues, immune deficiency diseases, or life-threatening conditions because the work is very comprehensive. Healing is more of a process, so I will try to take you step-by-step to manage your expectations for a healing journey that is more complex.

In case you're unaware, immune-related illnesses include more than three hundred different conditions, so they are much more common than one would think. You may easily be facing one or more of them.

If not, your body might *still* be in a state of decline; you might currently have multiple health issues or want to simply improve your quality of life as you age. You may even just be sick of taking all the pharmaceuticals you're prescribed and would love to have them reduced in quantity and strength. If any of these reasons sound familiar, this is a chapter to which you'll want to be attentive.

After reading the amazing success I experienced in finding the perfect answers to heal from so many different illnesses, you must now be asking, *what exactly did you do?* Well, besides how I strengthened my immunity, the big picture of the holistic healing process has not yet been presented in a step-by-step manner. That comes now.

A quick sidebar before we take the journey is a brief explanation of why I don't prescribe specifically and prefer to deal with process and simply opening doors. Each body is so unique that what worked for me in terms of treatment or therapy might not work for you at all. That is why a person must trust to be led to the perfect answer for you. My leukemia healing provides the perfect example of that.

I can identify a handful of methods that could be applied in the healing of this cancer successfully, since I've seen examples with other people. I chose high-dose vitamin C, but that doesn't have to be the case for someone else. I just happened to have been drawn to that method because of a book I'd read five years earlier that made an impression. In fact, it made such an impression that I used what I learned in that book to help my father extend his life significantly when he had inoperable lung cancer in the late 1970s.

Other than vitamin C, a person could use hyperbaric oxygen therapy; a pH program to elevate one's alkaline state; a diet based on the China Study information, which is predominately a whole-food, vegan diet; ozone therapy; Laetrile, and a few others. Many of these are used in combination with other protocols— like in my case, emotional healing, nutrition, and some lifestyle changes—but typically a person or his provider picks one of those and that's their focus, or you can pick a provider who works in the area to which you are drawn.

Also relevant is one's belief system, body type, and the way an individual person's cancer responds. People will be led to what works for them, so my information in this chapter is to give readers of glimpse of what a holistic healing journey looks like and the initial steps a person needs to take.

Now, back to the steps one takes on a holistic healing journey. My journey seemed to flow organically.

First, become determined.

Becoming determined is very different from simply wanting or hoping. Being bound and determined, digging in or being hell-bent are all ways to describe that strong, resolute, unwavering feeling one gets when you know exactly where you are headed and don't intend to let anything or anybody get in your way. I'm sure you all know that feeling, but if I didn't describe it well enough yet, this illustration might help.

Remember when as a child you defiantly stated, "*I don't care what you say, I can climb that tree.*" And you did. It was a knowing you had, and you proved to others you were right. Or, as an adult, when you struggled through eighteen-hour days, put your life savings into a business, and wouldn't give up because you know that business would be a success—and it was.

If you think back in your life, I'll bet you can find a time when you were that steadfast in making something happen—maybe through a sense of competitiveness, or maybe just some inner strength you didn't know you possessed. If you can remember such a time, take a moment to feel that again about your commitment to become healthy again. State your intention out loud. Don't say, "I want to get well," since that is merely stating a wish. Instead, say, "I am going to get well," or something similar. Say it and believe it—then let it go. A firm statement that is ambiguous about how you will get there or even when but is specific about the result. You will be heard. Then, you will be able to draw on that feeling again if you ever think about quitting.

Then, ask for what you want.

Some of you may have heard about *ask—believe—receive*; its often referenced when a person is seeking more abundance in their life. If you think the process is rooted in some type of metaphysical mumbo-jumbo, it isn't. In fact, even the Bible, in more than one passage, you will find very similar lessons. For example, in Mark 11:24, it says, "Therefore I tell you, whatever you ask for in prayer, believe that you have received it, and it will be yours."

This three-step process is so universal that it's hard to ignore. So, state what you want, knowing with gratitude it will somehow be delivered, and then turn it over. It's now out of your hands. Go on about your life and be open to the opportunities that present themselves—don't second-guess them because they will likely be Divinely led. And, as you will find, the Divine is always much smarter than you are.

This is how that worked for me when my husband and I had just left my rheumatologist's office in the early '80s. Remember the story? After my doctor recommended I take a mild form of chemotherapy called methotrexate for my RA. Remember, that's when I left.

When my husband asked what I was going to do next, I said emphatically, "I have no idea, but I'm not doing that. I'm going to get well." Emphasis on the "I'm going to get well." That started everything.

Even though I had no idea what I was doing next, it didn't matter. God heard me, the universe heard me, and my body heard me. Then, I let it go and had faith. There is no need to say that phrase over and over like an affirmation. Eventually the answers will begin to come into your life, as it did into mine—in the perfect order and at the perfect time. With each new interaction you will learn something new, so release expectations. You're no longer in charge.

Focus on the right thing.

I don't recall where I first heard the phrase "what you focus on expands," but the first time I heard it was like remembering something I'd always known. There are so many examples I could cite, but this one is the best. So, the question to ask yourself is are you focused on your disease(s) or your wellness?

My dear friend, Gladys Taylor McGarey, MD, MD(H), after decades medical practice and now retired and just past her 102nd year, shared this one with me years ago. Her stories have stories, as you can imagine.

She once was treating two women patients—both with lupus. One showed dramatic improvement, just like I did. The other woman couldn't get off first base. She was stuck with her illness and couldn't improve for the life of her. As hard as she tried, Dr. Gladys could not help this woman recover.

One day Dr. Gladys and woman number two were leaving the office at the same time. They both walked to the parking lot and parted as they walked to their respective cars. Dr. Gladys remembered something she had forgotten to tell the woman, so she turned to call out to her. At that moment, Dr. Gladys stopped dead in her tracks. On the woman's license plate was the word: LUPUS.

Now, Dr. Gladys knew exactly why this woman was not going to be able to find total healing. Here was a person who totally identified with her disease. She had not only accepted it—she was living it.

Put aside judgments.

I talk a lot about judgment because it's such a foolish exercise. In the scheme of things, we're just not smart enough to judge anything. We can have opinions, but hard judgments are another matter. In the case of health and healing, particularly so. It's easy to become judgmental when you compare one thing to something else with which you're familiar. Sure, they may be different, but that doesn't mean one is better than the other since appearances rarely have anything to do with the ultimate results.

In my case, I was initially judgmental of my first provider, my nutritionist. She worked from a home office, and back then (early '80s), I thought that was unprofessional. Ha! Instead, she was well-educated, brilliant, and totally focused on me. I felt I was the most important patient she had ever treated. She was the first to inform me that if my immune system was ever healthy, it could return to that state again with a little help. She also reminded me that all drugs either suppress or replace the function of the immune system—all of them. Within three weeks of a specific therapy and new diet, I noticed more energy and an improvement with my joint swelling and stiffness. My initial judgment was ridiculous.

Another case was when I was drawn into a dusty old health food store and met a beautiful young woman with a little girl voice (instantly, no credibility) who introduced me to a Rife machine I still use today, thirty-plus years later. This would be quackery to some, but it has been amazingly helpful to me. I love those two examples and, sorry, but I repeat them for a reason.

The illustrations could go on and on since I believe some alternative medical providers are just angels in disguise. They almost all are gifted in some way.

Act without fear.

"The secret to getting ahead is getting started." This is not a profound quote from a wise old sage, it came from the inside of a fortune cookie. I thought it was perfect. It takes many steps to complete a journey, and like I did to move forward, one must take the first step to begin. No fairy godmother with a magic wand will make healing happen for you; you will need to physically get out of your chair or off your couch and begin this journey yourself.

So, for those of you content to let a Higher Power deliver your miracle, I'm here to provide a reality check because God rarely works that way—again evident by one of my favorite stories.

A man was sitting on the roof of his house during a raging flood. He prayed and prayed for God to save him from the rising waters. During those prayers, a young boy floated by while holding on to a large log.

"Jump on," said the boy. "There's room."

"No, that's not too sturdy. I'll just wait here, God will deliver me," replied the man as he kept on praying.

Soon, the water reached the second-story window. By that time, a group of people came by in a rowboat. They yelled out to the man on the roof.

"There isn't much room inside, but you can hang on to the side—just jump and we'll pull you with us."

"No," the man said, "that seems risky. I'm praying to God to help me."

The water continued to rise and this time it was nearly to his chest. Soon, deep in prayer, the man heard a helicopter hovering overhead and saw a rope dangling from the open door.

"Grab on to the rope, we'll pull you up," they yelled from the chopper.

"I don't think I'm strong enough to do that," the man yelled back. "I'm in God's hands, and I know He'll save me."

The water continued to rise and finally the man became submerged and drowned. When he reached Heaven and came face-to-face with his Maker, the man cried out:

"Why didn't you answer my prayers? Why did you abandon me, God?"

"Abandon you?" God replied, "I sent a log, a boat, and a helicopter."

This story illustrates two powerful lessons. The first, how answers may come in ways we don't understand. It's not our place to judge, it is our place to have faith and take action. Second, to teach us that prayer alone is not enough if we don't do our part. Yes, to repeat another of my favorites: "God helps those who help themselves."

Throughout this journey, you must be willing to change.

Taking action often requires people to also make changes in their normal routines or normal ways of thinking. Change is not always easy, and most people avoid change because of fear—a whole chapter is dedicated to this subject!

Here are some common fear-based reasons for avoiding something like alternative care. "What will my friends think?" "My family will think I'm crazy." "I might fail." "I don't know enough yet." "It might hurt my image." "I don't know if I can trust them." "It's too risky." "Who knows how I might end up." "I don't have the energy" "I don't have any personal support." Replace the fear with faith and a sense of adventure! Most everything in this field carries less risk than conventional medicine's treatments, anyway.

In reaching wellness, you must let go of excuses and the need for validation from others. When something hasn't been working, you must have courage to let go of the same old same old. Maybe that's an overly stressful job, old ideas and beliefs, or unhealthy relationships. One of the reasons people don't heal is because they're afraid of the pain of letting go. Ask for the courage to let go of whatever remains harmful and ask for the strength to change to something more beneficial.

Realize when you need to become a priority.

Sometimes while recovering from a serious or chronic illness and while establishing new priorities and boundaries, you need to put yourself first!

I realize that may be a difficult step for the "pleasers" in the world. If you are one of those selfless people who give and give and give, find it uncomfortable to receive from others, and have a to-do list a mile long—that doesn't include anything that directly benefits you—then you may need to read and reread this section.

Making yourself a priority also requires an element of healthy self-esteem and self-love. By self-love I mean how much you value yourself and your life. That shouldn't be a stretch if you can remember that God gave you this phenomenal body as a gift, and all of us should try to honor that gift. I'll bet some readers are thinking that they *do* value themselves, but you'd be surprised how that isn't always demonstrated.

One classic example is one, again, shared by Dr. Bernie Siegel in his book *Love, Medicine & Miracles*:

> Consider, for example, Sara, a woman who came to me with breast cancer a few years ago; she was smoking when I walked into her hospital room. Her action clearly stated: "I want you to get rid of my cancer, but I'm ambivalent about living, so I think I'll risk a second cancer." She looked up sheepishly and said, "I suppose you're going to tell me to stop smoking."
>
> "No," I said, "I'm going to tell you to love yourself. Then you'll stop."
>
> "She thought for a moment and then she said, "Well, I do love myself. I just don't adore myself." (Sara ultimately did come to adore herself—and stopped smoking.) It was a good quip, but it exemplified an important problem many people have with

themselves. Self-love has come to mean only vanity and narcissism. The pride of being and the determination to care for our own needs have gone out of the meaning." (65)

We're reminded that thinking of ourselves first often makes total sense. Every time we fly, when the flight attendant announces that in the event of change in cabin pressure, we're to "grab hold of the mask and press it firmly to your face, pulling on the side straps to tighten the mask. Secure your mask, first, before helping any small children."

This, dear friends, is our ongoing reminder that if you don't take care of yourself, you can't take care of others.

You might need to learn to say *no* too.

In any healing journey, it's important to remind yourself often that you mean business in your commitment to self-care. If your body needs sleep, you must go to bed even if others are still up watching television. If you're hungry you need to eat, regardless of the time of day—even if others aren't eating. If your body requires certain food, you must be willing to fix yourself something different from what others around you are eating—without guilt or embarrassment. If you are overly stressed with a particular activity in your life, you must be willing to say no to participating—at least temporarily. Think of yourself first before you worry about making everyone else happy.

Now, I have earned the right to criticize individuals who rarely think of themselves first since I was a card-carrying member of the "everyone and everything before me" club. In my early years, I had the perfect role model to teach me the art of selflessness—my mother. She was a remarkable woman, who was considered by some to be the neighborhood saint. She cared for her friends, wounded animals, and the hordes of visitors who trekked out to Arizona for a change of climate. Her back door was always open. She sat and was patient regardless of what she still had to do or how poor she felt. She suffered the symptoms of her disease, also rheumatoid arthritis, in silence and always did for others without complaining and without caring for herself. She died twenty years too early.

Conversely, I knew a woman once whom I really admired as a mother. She had wonderfully behaved, happy children. And I asked her what her secret was in raising such a well-adjusted brood. Do you know what she said? "It's them, or me." Her response startled me because it seemed so out of character for her. But this loving, gentle, and compassionate woman had it right. She had household rules that included schedules for eating and sleeping so mom would have time to clean the house and take a bath. To her, that behavior wasn't selfish; it was simply a matter of survival.

Eventually there will be more than one resource.

As great as the first provider you find in the alternative space might be, what that person will share will only be part of what you will eventually need to heal. You needn't move on from them, but you can surely add to them to speed your recovery and expand your scope of knowledge.

I eventually ended up with a cadre of providers: first a naturopath, and then she was replaced by a holistic MD, and I added a chiropractor, an acupuncturist until he moved away, someone for colonics, a masseuse, and I was always receptive to a good book from one of the leading voices of integrated healing at the time. I saw them as I needed them, not in a routine fashion. Today, I have a smaller group and a couple of allopathic physicians, but my healing books are replaced by the most current podcasts, webinars, and profound emails that are forwarded to me. Well, today I write them more than I read others' work.

I also use essential oils and had my trusty Rife machine for diagnosis and treatment. Regarding that machine to which I was introduced in the back of the dusty old health food store in the early '80s, I felt a little better when I read in *People* magazine thirty years ago that mentioned in an article that Prince Charles and the Royal Family were into holistic medicine, took homeopathic remedies, and were devotees of several other alternative processes. A radionics machine was mentioned for diagnosing illness and diseases in their horses (they probably used it on themselves, too, but were too embarrassed to mention it in the article). The radionics machine is like a Rife machine. Now, as strange as it sounds, I used that machine for many things and still do today. It helps to reduce radiation after flying, boost the function of various organs, de-stress, control Candida, and detox, besides hundreds of other benefits. It has helped me dramatically over the years. It was one of the therapies I didn't tell anyone else about, except my husband, because my normal friends would have thought I was bonkers.

I had dropped all judgment by this time and regardless of how anything appeared, I took advantage of the opportunity placed before me. I found supplements to relieve my pain since I was going cold turkey without drugs of any kind and needed all the help I could find. I used meditation and became open, which I guess God understood and kept sending me winning methods to help.

In a complicated healing like to repair or reboot an immune system, it is never a silver bullet. It is always multiple options, so be open and willing and they will come.

Honor the coincidences.

As my journey continued, I began to treat my body with more respect. I welcomed all the information that came to help—books, tapes, and new acquaintances. I was open and I saw small amounts of progress with each step I took. There were no coincidences in my life; everything was happening for a reason.

As a good friend of mine once printed on the program for her wedding, because she and her husband had so many parallels to their earlier lives: coincidence is God's way of remaining anonymous.

Accepting a coincidence as providence takes faith, but recognizing that fact when it occurs is much easier. We all have said *isn't that a coincidence?* At some point, we begin to realize that they weren't coincidences at all. Coincidences are always Divinely inspired.

Welcome alone time.

Not surprising, when something like a debilitating or life-threatening illness hits, our priorities change. We're now *forced* to think of ourselves: how we hurt, how little energy we have, or what might happen as this condition progresses. Our families begin worrying about us, too, and often watch helplessly with how we're coping. If the problem is painful or debilitating enough, we can be faced with plenty of alone time.

If our condition is not life-threatening but we are just dead serious about plowing ahead to a healthier path in life, alone time will still become part of this journey. Alone time brings with it many benefits besides just the obvious healing time our bodies often require.

By carving out such time, you now can look at yourself, your health, your lifestyle, and your relationship from a fresh perspective. From time to time this is necessary, but for those of us who have continually pushed past logical assessment times in our lives, illness often forces the issue, and it's always beneficial.

Learning to go within and comfort ourselves is a very positive by-product of any reflection process and is a healing exercise all by itself.

Realize that old habits die hard.

All too often, when an immediate crisis has passed, we wind up going back to old habits, dropping the supplementation, and doing the same things we did before we became ill. That's not a good idea.

We all remember the definition of *insanity*: doing the same thing over and over and expecting a different result. That not only sums up the need for learning to embrace change—if we want a different result in our lives—it also reminds us that whatever change we initially adopted that brought about success, we should keep that in place and not go back to the old habits that caused our health issues in the first place.

Becoming ill forced me to stop my old patterns. During healing and decreasing energy levels, it was necessary for me to do less, so I began to make choices and select only the activities that were most important. I began to become more discriminating, and in doing so, it became one of the best benefits of my journey.

Time becomes your friend—not your enemy.

Time isn't something that you manage on this journey—it is what it is. Progress will also not happen on your timeline, so forget trying to control that either. With every visit, with every new treatment or remedy, and with every experience along the way, something new will be learned. The magnificent reality of a holistic healing journey is how the timeline gets set according to how quickly you and your body are ready for the next phase. You will have nothing to do with this timeline.

To completely heal, it could take weeks, months, or years. So, patience is a must. It's also important to remember how long it took for your body to decline to its current state. A body or immune system doesn't break down in a week or even a year. If your body took years of abuse, you can't expect miracles in a few short weeks.

Regardless of the timeline that will apply to your healing, be sure to give yourself credit on the journey and continue to have faith.

Gratitude fuels progress.

A little thank you goes a long way. Gratitude is an extremely powerful healing emotion that is central to accelerating one's healing experience. Living in gratitude is, unfortunately, not commonplace today. People simply move too fast to notice all the little blessings that surround them. They project into some future picture of perfection and therefore are never satisfied with the now. So, before you begin focusing on being grateful, you might remember to also crank your gears down a notch or two—in other words, slow down.

One great way to reduce the speed with which you are living is to meditate for a few minutes every morning to become more centered and to start the day with a more peaceful frame of mind. Sit in a comfortable bedroom chair, take a deep breath, smile gently, and relax. Meditation isn't as mysterious as it seems, and you may notice I've mentioned this multiple times in this book because it is such a healthy exercise. All this process entails is just sitting there with nothing on your mind and letting any thoughts that float into your head float right back out. If you focus on them, they will dominate your consciousness. Let them go, and if they are important, they return.

Once your mind becomes less active, you'll notice more that's happening around you and how time slows down too. You'll become more centered, grounded, and able to live in the present moment. Your awareness will become sharper, your appreciation will be heightened, and gratitude can't help but follow. A person can't be grateful for something they're too busy to notice.

When a person is grateful for the blessings in their life, life changes and more blessings seem to show up. That is a phenomenon that this simple story will illustrate.

Imagine one day you give your little niece a toy. The little one takes one look at the toy and throws it down on the ground. The next time you give the child a toy, she turns up her nose, drops it and walks away. On the third try, months later, with yet another thoughtful gift, this child doesn't even bother to open the sack for several hours; it just lies there on the floor. With an attitude like that, how likely are you to give that youngster another toy any time soon?

Conversely, you are friendly with the little neighbor girl who is delighted with the flowers you let her pick from your yard. She continues to thank you every time she returns for one more. On her birthday, a simple card from you brings a warm smile and a big hug. When you give her some of your junk jewelry for dress up, she squeals with delight, and the first time she wears it, scampers over to your house just to show you how pretty she looks. A grateful child is one for whom you can't wait to do more.

We are all children, in a way, and being grateful for the progress we make in our healing helps deliver more of the same. The more you are grateful for, the more will be delivered to you as your journey continues.

Chapter 13
EXPLAINING THE WORLD
OF ALTERNATIVE OPTIONS

Exploring the possibilities that exist outside the realm of conventional medicine can become an adventure if you allow it to be. In this chapter, I'll try to provide straightforward explanations of many of the alternative options that exist. In some instances, I've added additional color commentary. You'll note that the options range from those currently acknowledged by Western medicine to some of the lesser-known modalities.

As you read slowly through the list, you may be drawn to one or two of the options more strongly or become more curious about them. Those are probably the ones to which your body might be more receptive.

Acupuncture. Developed in China at least two thousand years ago, this method uses needles strategically placed on the body to open the flow of vital energy, or Qi (pronounced *chee*). This is believed to influence the balance of the body's natural health. Acupuncture is used for managing pain, relieving acute sinus infections, speeding healing of joint injuries, as an anesthesia in surgery and dental work, and many other specific conditions. Acupuncturists and practitioners of traditional Chinese medicine (TCM) receive certification after training and may be licensed in some states. Other alternative providers like naturopaths may also have training in this art. For thousands of years, people have seen relief by using acupuncture.

Affirmations. This is a therapy people can use to help reprogram their thinking and change the outcomes in their lives. Positive affirmations, written in the first person and in the present tense, are a form of autosuggestion in which the statement along with its desired outcome is deliberately meditated upon or repeated to implant that thought into one's subconscious. It is thought the most effective affirmations are those written then spoken with some element of believability. For example, if a person was grossly overweight, he or she would not say, "I am thin and full of energy," which would be an immediate disconnect to their subconscious. Instead, they might say, "I am becoming thinner and more energetic every day," which rings true with possibility. See the difference? This is easy to try on your own and without the expense of hiring a coach.

Acupressure. Also developed in China, acupressure is the older, original technique in the acupuncture genre. Acupressure is a Chinese home remedy to cure headaches, backaches, sinus pain, neck pain, eyestrain, and menstrual cramps as well as the pain of ulcers, and to help heal sports injuries, relieve insomnia, and alleviate constipation and other digestive problems. Many cruise ships recommend wristbands using acupressure to mitigate seasickness. This form uses the finger and hand pressure instead of needles to stimulate the Qi, the body's most basic healing energy.

As an example of how this is commercially applied and accepted, you may have seen recent ads on television for BeActive Plus, the acupressure system for instant relief from sciatic pain radiating from the lower back down a person's leg. This totally harmless method of treating sciatic pain merely puts pressure on a point beneath the back of the knee using acupressure. It is approved by the FDA as a treatment and is also very affordable. Acupressure works.

Aromatherapy and Essential Oils. The use of essential oils as aromatherapy can be documented in ancient Egyptian hieroglyphics and Chinese and eastern Indian manuscripts as well as the references in the Bible. These oils are primarily applied topically or diffused. It is believed these oils increase cellular oxygen, promote immune function, and open the subconscious mind, among many other things. Some use custom blends to alleviate fear, mitigate insomnia, and reduce pain. Practitioners vary. In the late 1920s, the name aromatherapy was officially applied.

Ayurvedic Medicine. This is a provider group that originated with the sages of ancient India five thousand years ago. This approach to physical health, mental clarity, and spiritual fulfillment was made popular in the United States by Deepak Chopra, MD. This practice is a total form of care and is best guided by an Ayurvedic physician, not because it's harmful but because it is complex. It treats patients initially by identifying the blending of certain body types with emotional tendencies, intellectual styles, and spiritual inclinations. That eventual identification creates a detailed portrait of each type of individual and is considered a holistic method of care. There is no licensing procedure and no accrediting board for Ayurvedic practitioners. Finding a good Ayurvedic doctor takes some effort.

Chelation Therapy. This a process by which chelating agents are administered to a patient that will bind with heavy toxic metals such as cadmium, lead, and mercury or others as well as minerals such as calcium so they can be excreted from the body. Chelation agents can be purchased over the counter and taken orally at home or can be administered intravenously under the supervision of a nurse, naturopath, or physician. There are over 150 doctors in the US that are certified by the American Board of Chelation Therapy. Some claim that chelation therapy may be useful to treat heart conditions, Alzheimer's disease, and autism spectrum disorder. However, I have no direct experience with this method except for taking Zeolite, an oral supplement, from time to time to help eliminate heavy metals.

Chiropractic. Started formally in 1895, this modality originated with the ancient Greeks in 1250 BC. It was the Greeks who first invented this technique by treating muscular and skeletal disorders through manipulation of the spine. Spinal problems can interfere with the nerve supply and blood circulation to the rest of the body as well as cause physical pain. This is effective for acute musculoskeletal pain, tension headaches, and recovery from trauma. Chiropractic therapy is provided by licensed chiropractors with the initials DC after their name. I've used chiropractic for decades. Choosing a chiropractor may be based on the techniques he or she uses since there are six or more methods of which I'm familiar. My chiropractor uses kinesiology to read my body, uses a block technique, and is highly intuitive, but others have other combinations of skills or schools from which they are trained as one may resonate better with your needs.

Colon Therapy (Colonics). This is also a treatment. A colonic is a form of hydrotherapy that gradually and gently cleanses pockets in the colon walls, rids the body of undigested food particles, and stimulates muscle tone. Such cleansing removes the debris that might be caked along the lining of the intestines and colon. My body responds after colonic therapy by demanding less food intake since nutrients are more efficiently absorbed after that process. Colon therapy is also used to relieve symptoms when lower back pain is aggravated by a distended colon. This therapy is also thought to help keep the colon free of bacteria since our diets today contain fewer stone-ground whole grains and high-fiber foods. Clinics associated with this form of therapy include the A.R.E. (Association for Research and Enlightenment—Edgar Cayce Foundation). Probiotics should be taken before and after such a therapy. Qualified practitioners are easier to find in larger, metropolitan areas.

Energy Medicine. According to quantum physics, as you go deeper and deeper into the workings of the atom, you see there is nothing there—just energy. If you can believe that, then this section won't seem so irrational. Energy medicine requires a complex explanation because its application is so varied. Techniques can range from Reiki healing, where one person uses his or her own energy or energy from an ethereal source to channel to the person needing healing; hands-on healing, more often associated with religious or spiritual anchored healers; to various machines including radionics machines, Rife machines, and more recently Energy Enhancement Systems (EESystem) technology, which uses custom-installed computers to generate morphogenic energy fields to promote healing and regeneration. This last system, as strange as it sounds, has been recognized at dozens of medical, scientific, and professional conferences around the world, and locations for treatment are sprouting up throughout the United States. The radionics and Rife Machines vary in style and quality, so research is necessary. Minerals and semiprecious gemstones also generate healing energy (each one is different).

As bizarre as some of these sounds, I've used an old Rife machine for over thirty years, wear a medallion and other products infused with EESystem energy for healing and energy enhancement, and carry specific minerals and semiprecious stones with me daily. I've had Reiki practitioners work on me as well. Since everything in our world is composed of energy, utilizing energy to heal makes perfect sense to me. This category is fun to research, and many other methods for energy healing exist, and you'll find that besides those I've not listed here, others will continue to pop up in the next few decades.

Feldenkrais Work. This is also a therapy that is a system of bodywork, movements, and floor exercises designed to retrain the central nervous system. This process is innovative, gentle, and quite effective in rehabilitating victims of stroke, cerebral palsy, trauma, and other serious disabilities. This can be an alternative to standard physical therapy.

Herbal Medicine. This practice treats disorders with medicines that are derived exclusively from plant materials. Practiced widely in Europe and the Far East, remedies are developed to suit each person's individual needs to help the body heal itself. You might find naturopaths, Ayurvedic practitioners, traditional Chinese medical practitioners, and holistic physicians, as well as some others utilizing this form of treatment.

Holistic Medicine. This is a provider group that includes MDs, commonly designated by MD(H), who believe in treating whole individual— the mind, body, and spirit of the patient. Patients are encouraged toward personal responsibility and are actively involved in their healing process. This modality is very open to alternative methods. There is a national American Holistic Medical Association (AHMA), which was cofounded in 1978 by my friend Gladys McGarey, MD, MD(H), who turned 102 in November 2022. There is no licensing requirement, but rather a common general philosophy about treatment and patient involvement. I was using this process intuitively in the 1980s before Dr. Gladys and I ever met.

Homeopathy. This is a provider group whose method of care was created in 1796 in Europe by a man who considered mainstream medicine irrational, largely ineffective, and often harmful. It was introduced to the United States in 1825. This system can be used with the help of a provider or through individual remedies one picks up at a health food store. As I mentioned before, this system of treatment is based on the use of highly diluted remedies made from natural substances that trigger the body's own immune response mechanism. Individual treatment remedies can be used for such common ailments as allergic symptoms, sore throats, postnasal drip, nausea, bruising and bone issues, bloating, food poisoning, bladder pain, and depression/grief, among so many others. Or you can seek the counsel of a trained homeopath to develop a constitutional remedy for you that will help with your physical, emotional/mental, and spiritual issues. Practitioners may be MDs, osteopaths, chiropractors, naturopaths, chiropractors, or laypersons. There is licensing for these practitioners in a few states. This has been the preferred method of care for the royal family for generations as mentioned in the last chapter. You will find medicinaries identified (the common pharmacy for homeopathy) or the designation for allopathic (conventional medicine) and homeopathic pharmacies throughout Great Britain and Europe. Homeopathy is a harmless form of care.

Hydrotherapy. A treatment that was first used by Hippocrates in the fourth century BC, hydrotherapy has been part of the healing tradition of nearly every civilization from ancient Greece and Egypt to Rome, where virtually all medicine was practiced at the public baths. Today, modern water treatments include baths, cold water sprays, rubs, steam inhalation, and hot and cold compresses. Internal uses range from enemas and colonics (detailed earlier) to drinking enough fresh, pure water every day to promote health. Spas provide some of these treatments, others may be prescribed by health practitioners.

Hypnotherapy. This treatment modality takes advantage of the mind-body connection by placing the patient in a hypnotic state to heighten suggestibility to affect relief or trigger a behavioral change. The best practitioners are inventive and willing to try new strategies to access spontaneous healing. Hypnotherapy can also be used in place of an anesthetic for surgeries or dental work or other direct healing methods that vary to help all facets of mind-body-spirit medicine. Only licensed hypnotherapists should be consulted for this modality.

Imagery and Visualization. This process of therapy has been considered a healing tool in virtually all the world's cultures including Native American tribes such as the Navajo and the ancient Egyptians and Greeks including Aristotle and Hippocrates. The power of "seeing yourself healthy" or specifically applying healing techniques in your mind's eye is well documented as effective. Imagery and visualization can be practiced in the privacy of your own home and with the aid of tapes or how-to manuals. No disease process is beyond the scope of guided imagery and visualization therapy for its potential is far reaching. Some people prefer to be led by a trained professional as in guided imagery. There are many books and videos on the subject so people can learn independently.

Juice Therapy. Another therapy can be composed of using fresh juices as a potent weapon against disease and such, by some, is considered a natural tonic. This approach offers a safe, inexpensive way to stimulate digestion, bolster the immune system, and encourage the elimination of toxins. This therapy is often used in conjunction with other natural techniques. You'll find Ayurvedic practitioners and naturopathic physicians to be the most likely to recommend this remedy.

Massage. This is perhaps the most natural of natural remedies. Touching your body where it hurts seems to be a basic instinct. Swedish massage is the most common form, formally introduced in the nineteenth century—although original forms of massage have been around for at least five thousand years. The benefits of this treatment include reducing muscle tension, stimulating or soothing the nervous system, enhancing skin conditions, improving blood circulation, promoting better digestion and intestinal function, increasing mobility in joints, reducing swelling and inflammation, and relieving chronic pain. Most everyone can benefit from routine massages—healthy or not. The only people who should avoid deep tissue massage are individuals who currently have a blood clot that is concerning. All states have licensed massage therapists.

Meditation and Relaxation. Relaxation and meditation techniques can boost immunity and lessen feelings of stress and anxiety. These techniques also reduce muscle tension, lower heart rate, blood pressure, metabolism, and breathing and spark tranquil feelings. You can do them in your own home, aided initially by tapes or how-to manuals. Most forms of meditation use a picture, a word (mantra), an object (such as a candle flame), or a sensation (such as breathing) to focus the mind. Others, like me, prefer gently letting extraneous thoughts flow through the mind (or immediately releasing thoughts without focusing on them) so the mind stays clear of useless clutter. The goal of such a process is to help a person become more centered, grounded, and able to live in the present moment, which also helps people feel less anxiety and stress in their lives.

Naturopathy. This is a provider group that relies primarily on reforming the patient's diet and lifestyle. Based on Greek, Oriental, and the old tradition of European health spas, patients find an emphasis on hydrotherapy, massage, and nutritional and herbal treatments. Some chiropractors are also naturopaths. These physicians, who generally have a ND or NMD after their names, may also use acupuncture, bodywork, and homeopathy and are effective as advisers and helping people design healthy lifestyles. NMD does not designate a medical degree but rather stands for naturopathic medical doctor, whereas ND stands for naturopathic doctor. Either is accurate, although the first is often misleading. Some states license these practitioners and in which case providers may also be able to issue a limited number of medical prescriptions.

Nutritional Therapy. This treatment therapy goes as far back as Hippocrates, who said in 400 BC, "Let food be your medicine and medicine be your food." This practice does not rely solely on your daily food intake and may augment therapy with supplements since much of today's food is processed or refined and loses its nutritional punch. There are also fewer vitamins and fiber, more fat, and more sugar along with food additives in many of today's foods, which can cause a variety of side effects for people ingesting them. Some foods trigger a weakening of the immune system. A good nutritionist or naturopath can help you find a nutritional program that suits your body type and metabolism and help you identify and eliminate foods that may be damaging to your health.

Osteopathy. This is also a provider group, and these physicians possess the same educational background as MDs but with additional training in spinal manipulation, such as acquired in chiropractic. Osteopathy considers all parts of the body. Cranial therapy is a specialized form of osteopathic medicine and is particularly beneficial for asthma, recurrent ear infections in children, sleep disorders, and other conditions rooted in nervous system imbalances. Licensed in all states, osteopaths can be differentiated by the DO after their name.

Reflexology. Although foot massages have been around since the beginning of time, this process releases stress and tension in the body by applying gentle pressure to certain areas of the feet. It started in the early twentieth century. The founder was American doctor William Fitzgerald, MD, and later mapped (on a foot diagram) by Eunice Ingham, an American massage therapist, who showed which spots on each foot to touch to aid healing elsewhere on the body. Practitioners can be certified by referral from the International Institute of Reflexology, the Reflexology Association of America, or by independent providers.

Regression Therapy. Also called past life therapy, regression therapy occurs when a patient is hypnotized by a licensed hypnotherapist who also specializes in regressions. The patient is then asked to recall past lives. This type of therapy can quickly and effectively resolve many emotional problems, conflicts, fears, and phobias usually in far fewer sessions than with conventional therapy. This specialty is one of the most recent and gained foothold in the 1960s.

Religious Healing. There are two basic forms of religious healing. The first is prayer in healing, which is supported by substantial research to support the beneficial effects of using prayer to heal. Belief on the part of the patient may be important; however, some research shows prayer to be effective even when sick people are unaware that they are the objects of prayer, referred to as intercessory prayer. Healing through the principles taught in the Christian Science faith has been effective for generations of Christian Scientists. Their form of healing is not faith healing, positive thinking, or self-hypnosis, but it is more complex in nature. Religious healing may also include hands-on healing delivered through Divine inspiration. Prayer and even hands-on healing know no denomination.

Rolfing. This form of bodywork attempts to restructure the musculoskeletal system by working deep tissue to release patterns of tension. Rolfing can sometimes be painful and is used to release repressed emotions as well as to dissipate chronic or habitual muscle tension.

Shiatsu. A Japanese form of bodywork in which the practitioner uses firm finger pressure that is applied to specific points on the body. It is intended to increase the circulation of vital energy. This can also be painful if administered by traditional Japanese therapists. The Western form is gentler.

Sound Therapy. About 2,500 years ago, the Greek mathematician and philosopher Pythagoras developed "prescriptions" of music to help his students work, relax, sleep, and wake up feeling better. Some believe the sounds we make with our own voices have even more healing power than external sounds. "Toning" sounds, self-generated, can help one relax, ease stress, and balance the body and mind. Today, sound is used to regulate heartbeat and ease pain. Some physicians use it to relax patients in surgery or during invasive diagnostic work.

Trager work. This is a gentle form of bodywork using rocking and bouncing motions to induce states of deep relaxation. This modality helps facilitate the nervous system's communication with muscles and is a particularly helpful rehabilitation therapy for people suffering from chronic neuromuscular problems, traumatic injuries, and many other disabilities.

Traditional Chinese Medicine (TCM). This provider group observes various parts of the body—especially the tongue and pulse—prior to providing treatment, which could include dietary change, massage, medicinal teas, and other herbal preparations. TCM can be highly effective for an extremely wide range of conditions from autoimmune diseases, including HIV and sexual deficiency, to chronic degenerative conditions including Crohn's disease and chronic fatigue syndrome.

Vitamin and Mineral Therapy. The practice of treating various conditions of the body with vitamins and minerals should be more accepted today since vitamin D, vitamin C, and zinc have been so widely acknowledged, especially recently. Such supplements are routinely used to replace vitamins or minerals that have been lacking for decades in a person's body. The bodies of some individuals also can become depleted due to stress levels, environmental pollutants, diet deficiencies, or for other reasons. I will caution readers that it is possible to create imbalances within the body with some minerals, so guidance is helpful. Additionally, many of non-water-soluble vitamins (such as A and E), if taken in too great a quantity, can become toxic to the body. It is best to have levels of vitamins and minerals tested periodically and to receive professional supervision from a naturopath, holistic physician, or other health care professional trained in nutritional therapies.

Yoga. This practice, which is believed to have originated nearly five thousand years ago, consists of breathing, stretching, and meditation and can take only a few minutes each day but is valuable for releasing built-up tension and stress. It is intended to join or balance the mind, body, and breath. You can take yoga classes or practice in your own home with the aid of books or audio and videotapes.

Chapter 14

FEAR IS THE ENEMY OF GOOD HEALTH

The quickest way to limit your chances of finding total healing is to live in fear. As simple as that statement sounds, it's quite a complex issue. Whatever your fear tolerance might have been in the past or your normal routine of jumping in and out of fear-based emotions in your life, the last three years put fear into a whole new perspective. Fear was non-stop and everywhere we looked. Folks might not have noticed what was happening, but I saw it clearly.

Yes, the COVID-19 ordeal was fear pollution on steroids. It engulfed most of the American public en masse encouraging everybody to be terrified of the unknown. That was a time when our leaders and the media, unrelentingly and continually, reported accounts of the spread of a virus that no one understood. We didn't really know if it was lethal, dangerous, or routine—but we were told it *could* be very bad. The implied threat hung over us continually as we were forced to stay home, cover our faces, avoid our elderly loved ones, and wait. It was the waiting and the uncertainty that made everyone more anxious and further exacerbated the fear.

I could go on and on about how the fear was fueled. We were told the therapeutics that maybe held some hope could kill us, how the vaccines would save—then later, maybe not—and that we had no idea where this thing came from or if something similar would ever happen again. We knew nothing for sure except how quickly COVID-19 was spreading, how hospital beds were overflowing, and to beware!

I won't take us through that dreadful experience again since we reviewed enough in the first few chapters, but what I did want to focus on was the damage that was caused by the fear itself. Forget the virus—this chapter is simply about the fear.

Our reaction to that fear, by not only the public but by our leadership, led to irrational and damaging action. It devastated our economy, made it impossible for small businesses to survive, set our children back educationally and socially, increased addiction rates, encouraged domestic abuse, kept people from much-needed medical care, escalated depression, affected the mental health of many—also in a negative way, and finally pitted one group of citizens against another harming friendships and family relationships. Our collective reaction to fear did all that.

The psychology of fear.

Fear is much more than a single emotion. "The environment created by fear in society can systematically produce more and more messages, stories and images that spread an even greater sense of threat, anxiety, and fear within any society. Every person responds slightly differently as some are more logical and tend to deal with such societal manipulation by not continuing to verify the information and confront it from a different point of view. Others are incapable of that and will repeat the ideas to others who are also receptive, reinforcing the fact that this all seems logical, familiar, and therefore believable." (66) Fear can become a movement.

Fear is such an easy emotion to stoke that it becomes a common tool to keep anyone, especially large groups of people, off balance and following orders. When a central boogeyman appears, be it a rival nation, a serial killer, or anything else we would normally fear—people tend to rally together and listen to their leaders about what to do next. This time, the coronavirus was the boogeyman.

To illustrate more precisely what I'm talking about, here is a medieval story that says it all. Once there was a man walking down a road into a city when he met Death. He asked her (Death) where she was going and why. She answered,

"I'm going to the city to kill a thousand people with the plague."

When the man arrived at the city, several thousand were dead, and not a single person was left alive. Returning on the same road, the met Death again and told her she had lied to him, that everyone in the city had died.

"I didn't lie," answered Death. "Exactly one thousand of the inhabitants died of the plague. Everyone else was killed by the fear of the plague."

Fear is insidious. It causes needless anxiety and stress, makes some people angry, and makes everyone who should be making good decisions about their health make bad ones. Fear can be deadly.

How do I know about fear?

There are a rash of fear-based emotions that people experience daily in their lives. Most folks don't even notice what they are. So, before I share a sample list of what fear-based emotions look like, I'll share a few I lived through.

The success of the business I started in 1973 was fueled by fear—a fear of failure and public humiliation, a fear of embarrassment, and a fear that I couldn't help a client who came to me with a failing little business. Thank goodness I wasn't angry or hateful, but I sure was resentful of authority, impatient, and continually worried. So, I've been there and done that.

It was my reaction to all those fears that led me to make horrible decisions about my lifestyle that eventually affected my health. That fear fueled the bad choices I made in relationships, kept me working nonstop for years, and kept me trapped in a form of medicine that was slowly destroying the remaining part of whatever healthy body I had left. The medical destruction over a twenty-year period (my twenties and thirties) I endured was primarily focused on the number of potent prescriptions I was given over those two decades as well as the lack of education about how I was running my health into the ground. My doctors, with more pills, enabled that behavior.

Yes, I understand fear and am not being judgmental about other individuals who reside in that environment. Instead, I'm hoping to educate others on how to recognize the signs of existing in a fear-based lifestyle and to help point in another direction before they end up with decades of health challenges to overcome just like I did.

My pretty impressive recovery from illness after illness starting in the mid-1980s could never have happened had I not learned to stare fear directly in the face. I think the first leukemia diagnosis was an additional launch point for me when I felt myself slipping into a fearful state again. After, as I mentioned before, wallowing in self-pity for a few days, I caught myself and said, *"If you want this to change, Sandy, you'd better do something about it."* I shifted from fright to fight.

It's amazing how becoming empowered by faith, or simply waking up, can make someone feel like David in the face of Goliath. That shift was not the result of some overpowering jolt of ego; instead, it was the blossoming of a quiet inner strength that made me realize that I could either lie down and take it or act! You know the one I chose.

When a person lives with too many fear-based emotions, it's exhausting, draining, and energy robbing too. The last three years of the aggressively promoted pandemic brought all that back into focus and reminded me that fear is truly the tool of evil.

What is the opposite of fear?

Most would assume the opposite of fear is courage, but that's not the case. Since fear weakens us and the love emotions strengthen us, could the opposite of fear be love? Another way to look at this is to ask what the opposite of love is. Most would say hate, but again that is wrong. The opposite of fear is love and vice versa. You'll see that all explained in detail as we proceed. If you are a religious or spiritual sort, it might make it easier to say that fear is the tool of the devil and love comes from God. That explanation is clear-cut.

I was so excited to begin this chapter because it's truly one of the most enlightening to me. If you are serious about keeping your immune system healthy, glance back at the chart and you will notice on the left it says (to avoid) fear-based emotions and encourages us to live (on the right) in love-based emotions.

This chapter includes a list, too. I've abbreviated the original list some so it would be easy to follow here, but there are actually subcategories under fear and then the list you will see here fall under each subcategory. It's the subcategories that make the fear connection easier to grasp. So, I'll try in narrative fashion to connect those points.

For example, on the original list, there were seven basic subsets of fear. Grief—when we mourn the injustices that were thrust upon us. In other words, an aversion or fear of accepting what is. There are ten specific emotions that stem from the overall category of grief.

There are also three more of those subsets under fear. Uncertainty—fear of the unknown. That one has eight specific fear-based emotions under it such as dread, doubt, anxiety, stress, and anxiety, among others. Abandonment—fear that we will not be accepted or will be ignored or forsaken. Five specific emotions fall under that one. Anger—fear of the unknown; that one has eight sub-emotions like rage, fury, bitterness, resentment, and aggression. All fear-based and all in the same family.

The same holds true with love-based emotions. All the wonderful emotions in that family stem from these much more love-infused categories: Happiness, Empathy, Certainty, Honor, Belonging, Wonder, and Acceptance.

Obviously, love-based emotions such as love itself, forgiveness, compassion, understanding, gratitude, kindness, humor, support, trust, and so on strengthen our immunity, and fear-based emotions such as fear itself, anger, resentment, guilt, hatred, impatience, greed, jealousy, worry, and so on weaken it. Does that make sense?

The reason I feel so strongly about this subject is because I have watched people make lousy choices resulting from an inability to think logically because of fear. Can you see how confusion and uncertainty could breed such feelings? If you can, it's then easy grasp how alarm, anxiety, apprehension, distress, hysteria, panic, and so many other emotions can result.

Instead of succumbing to such emotions, there are ways to control those feelings, catch yourself when you are slipping, and become more in control of your life so you can feel more confident (empowered) regarding the decisions you make.

Here are the examples of love-based versus fear-based emotions.

You can zip down each list and quickly identify emotions that are the most familiar to you—the ones you routinely call upon. The first is the list that stems from the emotion of love. These are all love-based emotions. So, it's easy to determine why God's language is so powerful and healing.

Affection	Amazement	Acceptance	Astonishment
Awe	Bliss	Belonging	Cooperation
Contentment	Comfort	Connection	Contribution
Caring	Confidence	Certainty	Compassion
Calmness	Composure	Delight	Dependability
Ecstasy	Euphoria	Excitement	Empathy
Forgiveness	Fortitude *(inner)*	Faith	Gratitude
Generosity	Helpfulness	Humility	Honesty
Honor	Humor *(innocent)*	Joy	Kindness

Happiness *(letting go of expectations and finding happiness in what is)*

Non-judgment	Pleasure	Peace of mind	Patience
Resolve	Relaxation	Relief	Respect

Pity *(not looking down on but seeing others and identifying with them)*

Sympathy	Self-control	Support	Surprise
Togetherness	Trust	Tranquility	Understanding

Unconditional love *(without strings)*

On the other hand, one could make the argument that fear is the language of the devil. Trying to elicit these reactions from another person is always negative and harmful. Yet, you'll repeatedly see this happen in families, friendships, and with society in general. It's impossible to read through this list and not sense how negative and destructive they can be.

Anger	Apathy *(lack of concern or respect for others)*		
Aggravation	Alarm	Abandonment	Anxiety
Aggression	Alienation *(separating from others)*		Apprehension
Animosity	Bitterness	Contempt	Depression
Competitiveness *(in other than sports or business)*			Disbelief
Contempt	Despair	Doubt	Disdain
Disgust	Dread	Distress	Dishonesty
Desertion	Distrust	Envy	Embarrassment
Frustration	Fury	Fright	Fear
Gloom	Guilt	Greed	Horror
Grief *(an aversion to accept what is or that things are wrong or unfair)*			
Hysteria	Helplessness	Humiliation	Hostility
Hatred	Hopelessness	Impatience	Isolation
Jealousy	Loneliness	Loathing	Neglect
Panic	Rage	Resentment	Regret
Remorse	Suffering	Scorn	Shock
Shame	Selfishness	Terror	Uneasiness
Uncertainty	Worry	Wariness	

I mean, really, can you see how much angst can be caused if a person constantly reacts to life in this manner? Conversely, looking back to the love-based emotions, how peaceful and calming those are. A much more comfortable place for your body to reside. More Heavenly, wouldn't you say?

Fear and love are mutually exclusive.

Since one emotion is the opposite of the other, fear and love cannot exist simultaneously. Therefore, if you're living with loved-based emotions like gratitude, compassion, or trust, one cannot be worried, afraid, greedy, or angry at the same time. It didn't have to be an opposite emotion of the one felt at the time, it need only be any fear-based emotion.

The goal is obviously to stay in the more positive, loving emotions so fear cannot surface at all. If a person has trust, faith, hopefulness, and gratitude about life and the many gifts they were given, it is impossible for even fear surrounding pandemics or epidemics to overtake them. A person can be aware of a situation without succumbing to it.

So, when you start your day, you have a choice. Do you begin it with gratitude, joy, and trust or worry, fear, and anxiety? Whatever it is, it sets the tone for how your day will flow and makes it easier for you to stay away from stressful situations and heal in love.

How fear can affect your health care choices.

Love heals, and fear does just the opposite. When we are operating out of fear, we make dumb decisions, listen to the wrong people, and end up weakening our own immunity just through the sheer emotions involved.

It's easy to avoid something you are either uncertain about or fear—alternative medical options often fall into the category of a subject many are uncertain about or fear. Alternatives may seem too fringy and not as solid as conventional and scientific medicine. That's normal because conventional medicine is familiar. Alternative methods represent the unknown. So, with something one knows little about, there are two choices for a reaction—learn more about it or run away. I've always been one to embrace adventure. Sound fearless? I suppose it is.

When people remain in their safe space, they like to say that conventional medicine is traditional medicine, but it is not. As I mentioned before, traditional means based on or related to tradition. Modern medicine, as we know it, only truly began in the twentieth century. However, acupuncture, Ayurvedic medicine, chiropractic, nutritional therapy, sound therapy, yoga, massage, hydrotherapy, imagery and visualization, essential oils, and other forms of alternative medicine have been around for thousands of years. It seems the tradition lies with the latter since all the near dozen modalities I've mentioned are still being used.

The longevity of these methods is unquestioned, and the reason they have lasted all this time is because they appear to work. Now, doesn't being reminded again about the history make the thought of exploring some of those options less frightening? Having more knowledge always reduces a person's fear.

Isn't everyone fearful?

Of course they are, but recognizing that fact is the first step to not letting fear control them. Again, Bernie Siegel, MD, from his book titled *Love, Medicine & Miracles*, focuses on the power of love in healing. In that one book, he talks about the three kinds of patients he experienced in his practice.

The first are the victims, who give up and die. The second are the 60 to 70 percent in the middle, who do what they're told, but rarely make hard decisions on their own. This group, he recounted, resists making radical changes in their lifestyles and are loaded with excuses as to why they aren't more aggressive about wellness. The third are the exceptional patients who refuse to play the victim to a disease. They educate themselves, they participate in their health care, and they demand dignity and control. They ask questions and are sometimes considered uncooperative or difficult as patients. They aren't afraid to make lifestyle changes and they are the most likely to get well. (67)

I would surmise the third group of patients are probably the first to use complementary methods to integrate into their conventional care or may select a totally alternative route if they get a doom-and-gloom prognosis. The exceptional patients Dr. Siegel identifies are not afraid to take action, and they accept risk as a means for ultimate reward.

The exceptional patients Dr. Siegel describes are the fearless ones.

Become empowered to overcome fear.

Since a couple of my conditions were chronic, I'd chart my progress over time so I'd recognize what was happening with the trend line. That personal knowledge provided a sense of control, so I felt less fear because I could track what was happening to me, and I could react on a dime if I needed to. I had some power in all of this. I could not only feel what was working, but I could see it reflected on the charts I'd made. Of course, not all people are as analytical as I have a tendency to be, but if you are also anal, make your own notes or charts. Sometimes just indicating when certain symptoms present on those one-sheet calendars with square boxes makes it possible to review easily and notice trends or patterns. Those tools will not keep you focused on your disease but rather focused on your progress.

I'd routinely bring my charts to doctor visits, not so the physician could review my hen scratching and try to figure them out, but after I noticed a pattern, I'd point them out. Sometimes they were important, sometimes not. I liked to understand the test results, too, so I'd always ask for copies and often an explanation. The more people participate in their own health care, the less fearful they feel.

Managing or eliminating fear.

Recognizing the fear when it happens is one thing, but staying in a fearful state is something different. The more you focus and submerge yourself in the fear, the more you can be assured it will dominate your existence. If you remember, after my first leukemia diagnosis, I allowed myself to wallow in a little self-pity and fear for a couple of days. After that, I recognized what a downer it was living like that, so I decided I wanted to get well, and in doing so I shifted into action. Action based on trust, faith, and fearlessness always breaks the cycle. The fear disappeared.

My situation aside, it doesn't matter why you're in fear, it just matters that you are. Many health-related reasons could trigger such a response. They could vary from receiving a lousy diagnosis and being uncertain what might happen next, facing a pandemic of God knows what that's spreading like wildfire, or even having troubling symptoms with no idea what those symptoms mean and putting off that valuable diagnosis. All these can automatically generate fear. Fear is normal. Staying in that place is not, and how you remain is up to you. These steps might help a person who wants to shake the fear and take control of their life.

Step one—don't make important decisions when you're overcome by fear. Nothing must happen in a split second, and making any rash decision is never smart. Depending on the situation, breaking away and allowing yourself to decompress is what is called for. So, you might take a few moments (or days) to regain composure, walk away from TV news temporarily if that is stoking the fear, tell your doctor you want to think about this for a day or two, or read up on the symptoms of your condition so you begin to recognize how many possibilities might exist for healing before your pre-imagined death sentence.

The key is to pull yourself out of the drama, quit focusing on the negatives, and don't allow those feelings magnify and magnify. What you focus on expands, remember? Pull away long enough to have a little chat with God or your Higher Power to ask for objectivity, good judgment, and more faith. Avoid making hasty decisions until you regain your objectivity.

Step two—realize there are two sides to every story and sometimes the story is shaped like an octagon with multiple possibilities or solutions available. The most obvious conclusion is not always the right one, which is why people are presumed innocent until all the facts are in. So, limiting final judgment, trying to gain a different perspective, and even inquiring about other opinions from people with more experience than you can all help. If doing a little independent research or seeking the counsel of people who have been successful in healing generally, something might resonate with you, and a new course of action could begin to feel right, logical, or possible. In other words, become open to possibilities.

Step three—shift to a love-based emotion and break the cycle. Again, remembering these two emotions cannot exist at the same time, if you are feeling fear-based, shift to gratitude. Just stop for a moment, look around with your eyes and heart open, and see the myriad elements of life for which you are grateful: that you are still alive, have a family you adore, a beautiful day, a pet you're crazy about, your spouse's support or talents, or anything in nature. If nothing else, do that, pause, and say, *"Thank God, I _____* [fill in the blank with something positive]." It could be anything from being financially secure, surrounded by lovely landscaping, living in a comfortable house to being blessed with great kids, loving grandchildren, or that pet you adore! It's easy to shift to gratitude, and that instantly stops the fear. Or you just could find something to give you a good laugh. Humor works magic, too.

Step four—learn to live in the present moment. Fear cannot live there either. Fear is rooted in the past or future. In the past, it's magnified by negative, old experiences. If you can replace those destructive feelings with a centered, present mind, it will keep fear away. A future focus opens the door to fear of the unknown. If you insist on projecting ahead in your day-to-day thinking, you'll find yourself in a state of worry, or worse. Replace that perspective with a realization that you only have control over what is happening this very second. That's it—anything in the past is gone, and anything in the future isn't here yet and could be subject to change. Staying in the moment allows you to choose your emotions here and now. Those are the only ones that matter.

Step five—smile more. It seems silly but it's hard to be hateful, angry, resentful, and all the rest with a big grin on your face. Besides, a smile and chuckle will release the tension brought on by seeing or thinking about something that would normally make you fearful. When you realize how ridiculous some of the games in life are, realize everyone faces health challenges and many overcome them through bizarre ways, and recognize that we all take this journey through life too seriously, fear vanishes.

Chapter 15

STRESS ISN'T THE KILLER—
IT'S OUR REACTION TO IT

Fear and stress go hand in hand. They're generally part of a vicious cycle; if a person is prone to living in fear-based emotions, he or she will exist in a more stressful environment. If a person lives with a mountain of stress, their reactions to that stress will cause additional fear and thus even more stress—as you'll soon recognize. Stress as everyone knows is harmful to our health.

This chapter is designed to explain how people react to the stressors in life, how we often manufacture more stress on our own, and how to avoid or get rid of stress altogether.

OK, stressors are everywhere. So, how do we keep from overreacting? My answer—by first recognizing what those overreactions are.

The most common reactions to stress.

The reactions to stress fall into three categories. You guessed it—those that are rooted in the physical, the mental/emotional, and the spiritual. Familiar categories because everything related to good health and healing fall into one of more of those categories.

First, there are physical reactions, which are the easiest to recognize. Some people overeat causing obesity and constant worry about their weight. Others drink too much, which might generate feelings of hidden guilt, pack on additional and unwanted pounds, or more likely add additional stress on romantic, family, and sometimes work relationships. Others become shopa-holics: "When the going gets tough, the tough go shopping." The latter reaction can often cause mounting debt and often guilt—two more stressors.

Some people suffer with insomnia fueled by worry, which robs them of needed sleep. Others become workaholics and bury themselves in a career or hobby to help avoid what is really causing the stress in their lives. Many self-soothe or medicate with drugs such as nicotine (smoking ciga-rettes) or overdo alcohol, take up or increase marijuana use, or resort to other drugs. The health results from any of those reactions can contribute to inadequate nutritional intake, direct weakening of the immune system (smoking/drugs), and other health issues exacerbated by the enhanced fear. Do you see how all of these could manufacture even more stress?

There are also mental or emotional reactions to stress, too, which contribute to more stress. Any of these will magnify any originating stressful situation: additional worry; overreacting, which magnifies the stressful situation; becoming angry; growing more impatient; casting blame; adopting stubborn behavior; being anxious; trying to over-con-trol; getting depressed; or freezing in fear. Every single one of those reac-tions will magnify the level of stress one is facing and often cause residual stress for others close to them.

People can react spiritually as well. The reactions of a spiritual nature can be the most damaging and cause even more devastating health conse-quences. When a person totally loses faith, feels completely hopeless, or gives up altogether, they can hasten the end of their life, as was described earlier.

Stressful situations are impossible to avoid since we're surrounded by them daily with issues as simple as trying to make a phone connec-tion with automation, repeated computer issues, or any technology that goes on the fritz. Do you react in anger, share the tale over and over, and continue to magnify a lousy situation? Or do you chuckle while you say, *"The hits just keep on coming!"* and go on with your day?

Sad statistics.

Once, on a practical side, we realize the damage stress can really cause in a person's life, it shifts this subject to one that carries a little more weight.

Just look at these stats: 75 percent to 90 percent of doctor visits in the United States are in some way related to stress. Thirteen percent of children will develop an anxiety disorder due to stress, and 49 percent of young individuals between eighteen and twenty-four experience high levels of stress from comparing themselves to others. There are even more statistics, but these three cover the age spectrum pretty well. (68)

For the eighteen-to-twenty-four-year-olds, the impact of social media magnifies their fear and stress levels. Those enhanced feelings include not being good enough to measure up, which can result in jealousy, depression, isolation, regret, self-loathing, shame, and a host of other fear-based emotions—because of comparing their lives to others. Social media paints everybody else's life as ideal, exciting, or romantic while these young adults live with less perfect bodies, faces, and lives.

The anxiety disorders of young kids are often a result of the environment in which they are raised or the lack of a home environment at all—resulting in abandonment issues. Emotions are powerful, stress is real, and fear-based emotions are at the root of much of it.

I hope readers are beginning to recognize that emotions and stress have a lot to do with our mental, physical, and spiritual health. I also hope this reinforces the concept of mind-body-spirit medicine and how we must value each element of this triad as equally important.

Prepare yourself to feel less stress, physically.

A person's body can feel stressed without the influence of any exterior stress-related factors. One reason could be a lack of vitamins, minerals, or nutrients, which could have been depleted by high levels of stress over the years. In that case, vitamin and mineral deficiencies can occur. One such example is when a person becomes anxious and the body goes into a stress response. At that point, B vitamins are drained from some organs and rerouted to others to compensate. This leaves fewer B vitamins left in the original organs for healthy functioning.

Vitamin C is also depleted when stress dominates, and that vitamin is essential for an efficiently functioning immune system. It's particularly important to remember this since, besides being the most powerful antioxidant that exists, vitamin C helps calm the sympathetic nervous system. Like the B vitamins, C is water-soluble which means your body can't store it for very long, so even constant levels of low stress cause a consistent deficiency.

A quick side story. After my first visit to Mrs. Kell, my nutritionist, and after she heard about the stress-packed eight prior years I had lived (no time off—remember?), she sent me home with a wonderful powdered and buffered vitamin C as well as B complex vitamins. Instantly after I took them, I could feel my body saying, *"ahh..."* It was a sigh that I heard internally that might be like how a person dying in the desert from dehydration might react after drinking his first glass of water. Or, when putting a soothing salve on a burn. This combination of vitamins instantly calmed my central nervous system so my body could relax. Soon after, I was tested and other supplements were added.

Stress also can decrease levels of vitamins A and E as well as calcium, magnesium, manganese, and zinc, plus other nutrients like proteins. Also, since stress produces increased amounts of cortisol (the stress hormone), this factor alone can also decrease the expression of vitamin D in the body. So, excess stress can cause the suppression of vitamin D synthetization as well. Remember what strengthens our immunity? Many of those very vitamins, so simply living with constant stress, or generating your own stress daily, depletes your body of needed nutrients to stay healthy and function normally.

Now, if you don't live a stress-filled life, you may still be deficient having been born that way. The stress the mother felt during pregnancy the unborn baby also felt. There didn't have to be sudden trauma for one's mother—there could have just been constant low levels of stress from worrying about finances, personal insecurity, a challenging relationship with a spouse or other family members, and a host of routine stressors with which some people don't effectively deal—or surely emotional issues causing a constant stressful state.

In my case, both were contributors to the deficiencies that were apparent in my body since I continually presented with these emotional symptoms—I often felt out of control, jumpy, and more irritable or impatient than someone else with the same type of lifestyle. These were all signs my central nervous system wasn't balanced and calm. Friends would just describe me as a Type A personality, but it was more than that. I completely shifted my temperament (maybe not my speed at accomplishing things, but surely my attitude) when the right level of supplements was added.

The goal is always to keep our bodies in a peaceful state so the rest of our lives can flow that way, too, but nobody can exist today without suffering the effects of too much stress in work, relationships such as marriages and divorces, raising children, surgeries, accidents—heck, simply living life. I'd guess everybody is deficient in something that if added back into their daily routine would make a positive contribution to the way their body functions and the state of their overall health. At least, that's one place to begin.

Conventional medicine is weak in this area. It just isn't in their wheelhouse which is why they often rely on recommending the basic daily requirement found in a multivitamin, which is not close to being adequate. I'd recommend people who are taking a multivitamin just save their money and put the same funds to specific nutrients in which they are lacking. Targeted supplementation is always best; take what you need, not what might be good for you because the list of the latter is endless—and needlessly expensive.

Identifying intolerances that stress your immune system.

One can have internal stressors that are subtle and that we don't notice—however, our immune systems might. This one is a huge issue, and for anyone suffering from a chronic illness or autoimmune or immune deficiency disease, this one single issue could really make a difference once corrected.

Intolerances, which cause such stress, are different from full-blown allergies, which might result in hives, headaches, or other common symptoms. The reactions to intolerances are more subtle but strong enough to pose stress internally to your immune system. Because it tries to cope with the intolerance, the efficiency with which it routinely functions is diminished dramatically.

My sensitivities happen to be gluten, sulfites/nitrites, and pork. If I eat any of them (even minute amounts), even today, I can end up RA pain—within thirty-six hours—in one of my joints that can last several days. Just enough stress to push my fragile immune system over the edge. So, I don't risk it. Pain is a great motivator.

There are basic rules governing the phenomenon of intolerances. Most people facing immune issues have one or two serious intolerances of which they aren't even aware. There are a couple of ways to identify what those might be.

Many people simply crave their poison so it's easy to identify the substances on which addictive/compulsive personalities tend to binge or become predominant in their diets. You can identify that substance or substances yourself by adopting a simple basic diet of basic proteins and green vegetables for a week and then adding back foods at three-day intervals—starting with those you eat most frequently. Within thirty-six hours, you should notice reactions if they exist.

A quicker way may be to eliminate one of those commonly dominant foods for a week to ten days and see if you notice symptomatic improvement: inflammation, bloating, pain, headaches, foggy headedness, irritability, and so on. It doesn't have to be a food. It could be the method of processing a certain food or a drink that contains something your body reacts to. For some, diet sodas even cause weight gain, so your issues don't have to be those as obvious as strawberries or chocolate. Don't look for an immediate reaction because food intolerances can show up as far ahead as the thirty-six hours I mentioned.

If you don't want to attempt this alone, a good nutritional counselor, coach, or perhaps someone in your holistic physician's office can help. Intolerances don't show up routinely in skin testing or blood testing, the common form of allergy testing by medical doctors, although allergies would.

Old stored emotions exacerbate stress too.

Here's one quick way to see if this section might apply to you. If hot buttons exist with a parent, spouse, friend, or others with whom we are close—even someone in the workplace—you know the trigger that causes you to react. We've all had such experiences when we've blown up over something insignificant and wished we hadn't.

If you are someone who doesn't like being out of control or reactionary but can't put your finger on why this happens to you, this explanation might help. Perhaps you snapped back at a friend who said something innocent that just hit you the wrong way. Was it your friend's fault? Or yours?

Unless it was overt and malicious, it was your fault and was cause for one of these three reasons. First, because this person has done the same thing over and over and you've never dealt with the situation effectively before. There's an immediate lesson there, to try to solve problems when they occur, not store the feelings away.

Second, because you just had a lousy week yourself with a variety of things bothering you with which you haven't effectively dealt, and they mounted one on top of the other. Your stress level was mounting, and your friend was just the tipping point so he or she got the reaction for all the week's madness.

Finally, it could be what that person said that triggered old emotions from the way you were treated as a child by a parent, for example, and you never dealt with those feelings effectively either and they've been tucked away in your emotional warehouse for decades.

We aren't supposed to overreact in life. Still, people are human and many people stuff and store their negative emotions, bury them down somewhere and don't effectively release them. That habit is very unhealthy in the long run.

What makes people stuff and store emotions?

I believe the most common reason for stuffing and storing is to avoid dealing with stressful problems. If you are afraid of unpleasant interactions and don't confront anyone, perhaps because you don't have the verbal tools to handle the situation easily, there are answers for that.

The easiest method is to approach the person with love and a question about how the two of you might deal with this issue or how they might help you deal with an issue that specifically upsets you. Avoiding words that blame them, identifying their actions, or using "you" words in relation to them also helps. In any such discussion, it's best to focus on your feelings, not their actions. The more humble, vulnerable, helpless, and loving you can be is also helpful. At the very least, you can pray for a little Divine assistance with your approach and hope for the best. If your intention is loving and pure, odds are the result will be positive.

What are the excuses people use to stuff and store?

This is how people internalize excuses to keep from solving an uncomfortable issue in the first place. They initially can make one of these excuses to themselves while they are stuffing and storing the negative emotion they felt. After the first time or two, it becomes habitual and no excuse is needed.

The first method of avoidance is to minimize the experience and excuse it away, so they don't have to deal with it. That response is also called enabling. They minimize bad behavior or harmful behavior from the other person allowing it to continue because they are either afraid, don't have the tools, or don't want to deal with it. They enable the behavior to continue.

Another common one is to procrastinate with the issue, saying to yourself that you will take care of this another time and then never get around to it.

Still another is to give in to fear by thinking this issue can't be dealt with without causing even worse problems. The fear of addressing the initial issue makes the fear much greater in the long run since avoiding a potential solution becomes the rationale.

Then, there's the ostrich approach. A person could also simply play make-believe and deny the event ever happened—to others and to themselves. Never talk about it—never deal with it or even think about it. That never works either in the long run.

Finally, walking away from the relationship or situation or even quitting a job is a radical but often-used method too. That is having such a lack of emotional maturity that dealing with any emotional issue is almost impossible for that person.

Can you imagine how draining that could eventually become to a body that has to hold in those uncomfortable or even painful emotions for years or decades or even life? Each avoidance and the routine stuffing and storing of the emotions related to little things, big things, and sometimes life-altering events fuels much more damaging emotions in the long term like uncontrollable anger or rage. It can also result in physical illness or pain.

One quick side note. One of my friends just read a book by John E. Sarno, MD, titled *Healing Back Pain: The Mind-Body Connection*. His book explains his theory of tension myositis syndrome, a condition that causes real physical symptoms (such as chronic pain) caused by psychological stress, not pathological or structural abnormalities. My friend has stuffed and stored for decades, and one reading of this book has given her the tools to eliminate her chronic shoulder, mid-back, and other related pain that has become increasingly unbearable in her later years. She's a smart one, understood what she read, and applied the parts that resonated with her. So, see? More proof that stuffing and storing is harmful and can result in physical symptoms too.

How can we tell if we've held on to an old, negative emotion?

When we hold on to old childhood or other emotions that we stuff and store, it makes living a relaxed, peaceful life impossible. It's easy to tell when you are holding on to old stuff. These are a couple of the signs. When you have a sensitive, old relationship or situation and you bring it up routinely with others—if you find yourself getting worked up, your voice getting louder, becoming more animated, or noticing the fact that you can go on and on and on about it—these things all indicate you've never released it.

If old situations pop into your head from time to time that were unpleasant, that's your body reminding you to deal with those too.

There are many ways to release stored old emotions. If you believe that might apply to you, find a smart coach or counselor with whom you can confide and who might be able to help. There are some fascinating alternative methods for clearing old stored emotions or simply reframing them that can be accomplished in one or two visits. Ask people who might know, or do a little research yourself. Once you rid yourself of those unhealthy emotions, your ability to manage stress will improve.

You can also limit the new stressors you experience.

Again, it's not a heavy lift if you recognize what those new stressors might be.

Step one—listen to your body. Try to remember some of the signals your body will provide when you're in a stressful experience. Notice when you feel those signals, and temporarily remove yourself from the room or situation. If you're living within a constant environment where you receive these signals routinely, learn to alter your routine so you can take a walk or go for a drive to gain perspective and release some of the stress. A break and time out, always helps calm the waters before trying to solve the issue, which is the overall goal.

If something is too loud around you and is stressful, your body wants to (and sometimes does) duck or cover your ears with your hands. That's protection and a signal to move out of hearing distance.

Toxic smells that make you run away, again, a normal body response to which you should promptly respond, or your immune system will overcompensate and become stressed as a result. Plus, all the others we mentioned in earlier chapters

Step two—watch yourself. If your own stress-generating behaviors and attitudes are causing you more issues in your life, you can correct those too. Here are a few self-imposed stressors: perfectionism—if that is one, learn to delegate. Insisting on doing everything yourself won't leave you much time for the fun things in life. A friend who couldn't bear watching her cleaning lady not approach each task exactly as she would finally learn to grab her bag, jump in the car, and do something outside of the house when her cleaning lady was there. She didn't have to witness a different cleaning method than one she used (while it was happening), but she always returned home to a clean house.

Controlling behavior—in this case, learn to see the big picture and let go of details. Controlling others is a futile exercise that's simply exhausting. Most of us can't control ourselves, let alone anyone else. Remember, fear is the driver of control, so replace fear with gratitude, appreciation, or another emotion that helps you let go of the grip you have on others.

Step three—your own lack of self-esteem could be generating your stress. If you won't speak up for yourself, won't set boundaries and limits for others, and if you aren't on your own priority list—all these are possible to change once you recognize the issue might exist.

Step four—quit overscheduling your life. Most timelines we set for ourselves are arbitrary. If you don't adjust, sometimes life will intervene with an illness or crisis that stops you from pushing ahead on your list of to-dos. Making the adjustments yourself is much easier than waiting for the earthquake to occur that stops you.

Step five—clear the clutter. All matter is energy, and the more stuff that's stacked or strewn around the more energy it generates. Order is more peaceful and more calming. Wonder why monks live in sparse surroundings? It's not just to exercise sparsity, it is also more calming. Try cleaning up or tiding up one space (desk) or one room. You'll be amazed.

Step six—set limits and boundaries. Learn to say *no*. Just that little exercise frees up time and allows you to breathe and relax. Life will flow at a calmer pace.

Step seven—stop rushing. The tendency to rush isn't always a voluntary choice; sometimes it is an involuntary part of being deficient in the right supplementation of nutrients. Additionally, slow breaths, living in the present moment, and learning to clear your mind also help. Rushing manufactures stress. You can get rid of tension by eliminating your tendency to rush. Pace your life more effectively, get up earlier, or start out to a meeting earlier. Being a victim of the clock is a habit. When you slow down your pace, time will slow down too.

Step eight—stop worrying. This one is the worst. As was stated before, worry comes from not living in the present moment, stressing over the past (things you cannot change this second), and worrying about the future (which isn't even here yet—and the situation could completely change before then). Your power is in the *now*. Worrying about what someone else will or will not do is also a waste of energy. Others are impossible to control, and sometimes it's better not to know the detail of everyone else's thoughts and actions.

Another solution for constant worry is to "let go and let God." Give your problems over to someone else: angels, or even inanimate objects as some cultures do with their worry beads or dolls. They assign a worry to each bead or doll and then forget it. Simply say, *"This is too big for me to deal with, it's now in your hands."* I do that often with God. He is much better at everything than I am. I certainly don't second-guess His capability by worrying about what He'll do with the situation.

Step nine—learn to live in the present moment. Although I alluded to that in the paragraphs above, learning to meditate will help you stay present. Meditation is simple; it's just a matter of not holding on to thoughts that flow through your mind throughout the day. Stay focused on what is before you and ignore everything else, even what might be passing through your mind. We only hold on to things because of fear— we might lose the thought. Instead, I simply have adopted the belief that if the thought is important enough, it will return. If it doesn't, it was a waste of my time anyway.

Effective stress reduction techniques.

There is no need for much detail on these since many are self-explanatory. Here are a few suggestions. Meditation, exercise, experiencing quiet time to relax and decompress, and creating a few affirmations for strength and insight. Affirmations that have a believable ring to them work better than ones that are complete fantasy, as I mentioned before.

Deep breathing, guided visualization to relax—there are plenty of sources to find those and prayers to find strength and insight. Instead of praying for a situation to go away, pray for the strength to deal with it or the insight to better manage it with grace and dignity.

One of my favorites—find humor in situations and lighten up. Don't take everything so seriously or personally, even if someone is calling you names or accuses you of something you didn't do. I see that a lot in politics, and always remember, projection is a common intimidation technique. People often accuse others of things they're doing themselves. It's like the person doing the accusing is holding a mirror directly in front of where they are, and they're really talking to themselves. If you can picture that occurring, it helps.

My very favorite—find a spiritual connection that comforts you. There are so many options here: join a church or some way to commune with others in worship; connect with your angels; read spiritual books; hang with like-minded friends; journal to help clear your mind; meditate—I can't stress the power of this enough; ask for solutions and then be open to what comes; and finally, find comfort knowing those you love on the other side really aren't that far away; some people find great comfort in knowing that love and support exists.

I read a book a long time ago titled *You Are the Answer* by Michael J. Tamura, who was a gifted spiritual adviser and healer. At one point in his life, he asked the universe to help him become lighter in spirit—not so dense and heavy. More joyful, spiritual, and elevated. What he didn't recognize is that he'd be given circumstances that were anything but *light* so he could practice becoming all the things he asked for help with. Sometimes God helps us in ways we don't immediately recognize.

All the stress you wish would evaporate in your life might begin to dissipate once you quit stuffing and storing the stresses you encounter, stop manufacturing your own stress, help your body better cope with the stress that's unavoidable, learn to avoid stressful situations, and release the reactions to stress you've hidden away. If you begin to take on a couple of those suggestions, who knows, suddenly you might end up with a more peaceful life, and all the time it was up to you.

Chapter 16
CONNECTING THE DOTS

There were many points covered in this book, so maybe a little post-read analysis will help you refocus on the elements that will be most important for your health going forward.

I started this book with a candid look at the last three years, since that period had defined characteristics and a finite timeline. A great period in which to take a closer look at the leaders who manage our nation's health care. The greatest lesson from that period might have been that conventional medicine, the system of care we thought was beyond reproach, isn't perfect. The institutional leaders and the institutions that govern our system of medicine aren't perfect either. The COVID-19 pandemic brought all that into focus. So, in hindsight, it should now be acceptable to acknowledge those flaws, to analyze them in retrospect, and even to criticize them if we see fit. Why not? It was our bodies, our health, and our lives that were being affected by all the decision-making. Of course we're entitled to an opinion.

Some of us also noticed the inconsistent directives, the knee-jerk reactions, the government overreach, the massive egos on display, and the tendency for people who are in control to simply want to grab more. We also noticed a lack of transparency and all the questions that remained unanswered. We were taught to fear this virus because we knew little about it—except that it spread quickly. Our individual power vanished, common sense flew out the window, and we were all intimidated into silence. It was the government health care bureaucracy and the pharmaceutical industry who were in charge. Maybe we can now recognize the fear that was emerging.

While we were left to wonder why clinical frontline physicians were ridiculed and silenced, in this book we learned more about how vaccines functioned back in the old days and how they appear to function now. While isolated during the pandemic, we hopefully began to see that COVID-19 brought with it two major blessings: the immune system was finally acknowledged in having some role in our preventive care and that simple supplementation with vitamins and minerals might help strengthen our immunity to make us all healthier. Maybe common sense entered the picture here, too.

Although many ignored the nuanced message stemming from the two blessings that surfaced, I heard them loud and clear, and this was the impetus for this book to further empower readers. I hoped you would all learn more about the magnificent bodies we were given, why our immune systems are so critical to good health, and what we can do to keep it healthy and in perfect working order.

We might really have power over diseases after all!

Prevention and personal responsibility were highlighted.

The subject of prevention took center stage in this book since it is a subject that rarely surfaces in doctor visits, and if it does, it's so cursory that we blow it off. Instead of thinking prevention, we run to the doctor with every little ache and pain demanding antibiotics or other pills to give us a quick fix for what ails us. We've abdicated personal responsibility because that's been enabled by our health care system and insurance industry. We've become a society that overmedicates, which data proves, and that may not have been a smart choice.

We also learned that we don't live that long compared to other countries, with the most impressive country living more than six years longer. We also realized how hypocritical it is for institutional medicine to ridicule most natural or alternative forms of care because it is in those environments where preventive care thrives.

In addition, we learned how much power the pharmaceutical industry wields in our system of medical care and how the enormous amounts of money everyone spends on pharmaceutical drugs has not necessarily helped us become or stay healthier as a nation.

We learned that our doctors aren't educated about preventive care, so they aren't equipped to educate us on how we can help ourselves. We learned there may be safer and just as effective methods we could employ first before more radical treatments are accepted, and we also learned that when we hear a bad prognosis that it's perfectly fine to ignore it and still look for answers.

If nothing else, perhaps we learned that—as my history attests—answers might exist outside of the world that most of us were taught was the only place to look, and that our personal responsibility is a paramount factor in living a healthy life.

What has happened to life expectancy the last two years?

The longevity we reported prior took us through the beginning of the year 2020, or rather the end of 2019. What about the last two years?

As you'll see, the news is not good. Not because of COVID-19 since the world faced the same virus. Still, the United States continues to disappoint—and as we see this current data presented in an article from the Council on Foreign Relations with data from the CDC, clearly not sources outside of the controlled narrative, the US continues to look dreadful.

"The last two years marked the biggest drop in a century, with life expectancy sinking to 76.1 years for Americans born in 2021, according to provisional data (PDF) from the U.S. Centers for Disease Control and Prevention (CDC). This is down from an average of around 79 years in 2019, an enormous difference considering health experts typically measure life expectancy shifts in months, not years." (69) Our earlier chart pegged our life expectancy at the end of 2019 as 79.11 years. Apparently, now it has dropped by three years in a mere twenty-four months.

The above article continued: "Despite being a top spender on health care, the United States is an outlier among its peers on life expectancy. It sits well in the bottom half of countries in the Organization for Economic Cooperation and Development (OECD), a grouping of several dozen mostly high-income nations." In this group Japan was the highest, at eighty-five years, and the Central African Republic is the lowest at fifty-four. Still, many countries that are poorer than the United States have higher life expectancies. (69)

Although this source ranked only two dozen high-income nations, the chart I quoted earlier included over 190 countries around the world, so in this latter chart, Japan was ranked first when it was second in the earlier one with Hong Kong being first. Other differences in ranking were only due to additional nations being recognized, and where they fell, the longevity stats were not affected by the number of countries being compared.

Continuing from the same Council on Foreign Relations (CFR) article and quoting the CDC in attempting to credit our decline in life expectancy to vaccine hesitancy, its conclusion is inconsistent since, as the article goes on to state, "Increases in deaths due to the coronavirus disease accounted for just over half of the decline, according to the CDC … but the CDC found that also higher was mortality due to unintentional injuries and heart disease, among other causes. The rise in unintentional injuries was driven by drug overdoses, as COVID-19 has exacerbated the country's opioid epidemic." (69)

Because this is such a serious issue, I'll make one more reference to this article when they say, as I pointed out earlier, "'The broader deterioration in Americans' health worsened the toll of the pandemic in this country, with higher rates of cardiovascular disease, obesity and diabetes leading to more COVID-19 deaths than many other peer nations,' as CFR S Thomas J. Bollyky says." (69)

I ask readers to reflect back on two key points. First, if we were a healthier society, without the propensity toward cardiovascular disease, obesity, and diabetes, which does not plague all other nations, we might have withstood the COVID-19 crisis without as many deaths, as other countries did. And second, how many of the draconian mandates forcing isolation, lockdowns, and business closures might have contributed to the death risks caused by addiction, postponed medical treatment, and depression?

Nothing is simple, but the data speak for themselves, and it is clearly time for the American people to start making their own decisions, take more personal responsibility for their health and quit relying solely on the pharmaceutical industry to solve every health issue we face today or that comes in the future.

Individually, we have more power over our health than you might imagine.

A few more dots to connect.

The security of our good health lies with the most important tool we will ever have in the healing process—our bodies. Lessons about how to strengthen our immune systems, how living in fear weakens our immunity, and how we should learn to recognize, avoid, and release stress is critical to good health. Beginning to understand what alternative options look like and their impressive histories will also, hopefully, take away some of the mystery. I hope readers will begin to realize the mind-body-spirit connection is powerful. Most importantly, that anything is possible!

For those readers who actively practice their religions, the spiritual side of healing wasn't much of a lesson, but for the rest of the readers, how even the simplest spiritually related emotions like totally giving up, feeling hopeless, and accepting victimhood as an absolute are horribly destructive. On the flip side, how hope, trust, faith, and of course love open doors and heal in miraculous ways.

Answers for healing can lie in the most obvious places, even within our daily emotions, the simple choices we make to our lifestyle and the attitudes we choose to adopt. Yes, we have enormous control in the kind of life we choose to lead—one that's on a path to healing or one that traps us as a victim of illness. We always have choices, and we are the ones who can change a dreadful life into a joyful one.

I believe my own examples of healing may have opened a few eyes to what benefits there can be to becoming open, trusting more, and having the courage to follow where we're being led. Perhaps we learned that our intellect isn't the end-all and that our gut might produce just as much wisdom. That intuition may be just as powerful as we've been taught our minds are.

Simple and natural remedies often work, and finding very basic solutions for some of the health risks people face could remove some of the dread around the simple word virus. If your immune system is strong, regardless of your age, you will have fewer comorbidity issues and therefore become less susceptible to all forms of viruses and illnesses that exist today.

Although I tried to make this book rich in content and one to which you will refer back for additional support, there's still something else you should know.

Illness can be a gift.

More than a simple glass half full or half empty analogy, the fact remains that many illnesses bring with them gifts. Sometimes illness is our teacher while providing us time we need to reflect on issues that could improve our lives as well as perfect the growth of our souls. Often illness points to an issue that could improve the quality of our lives if we address it—evident when we track the emotional root cause of a particular condition.

Other times illness merely provides that much-needed time out for our own self-reflection and emotional healing. Alone time is healthy, and illness frequently gives us plenty of that—especially when a person faces chronic or life-threatening conditions. That solitude provides a chance to think through relationships that need mending, forgiveness that needs practicing, spirituality we've lost touch with, and how much more we could appreciate and learn to love ourselves.

Here is a fascinating list from a classic best seller titled *Getting Well Again*, which features revolutionary lifesaving self-awareness techniques from decades ago, by O. Carl Simonton, MD, Stephanie Matthews-Simonton, and James L. Creighton. When surveying their patients, they found five categories of benefits that seemed to be the most frequently listed when asked how their illness benefited them.

See if any of these have ever applied to you—or currently apply. Be honest with yourself, and even if you can relate to some or most of these, be kind to yourself when the realization hits you.

1. Receiving permission to get out of dealing with a troublesome problem or situation in your life.

    This can be permission to hide and to avoid dealing with something uncomfortable or something with which you don't yet have the tools to deal. With the gift of the time you need, you can often strengthen yourself in that area of life where you are more vulnerable or not as well equipped.

2. Getting attention, care, and nurturing from people around you.

This is a much more significant statement than it appears because besides providing the opportunity to gain attention, care, and nurturing from others, it also could be providing you the same opportunity to gain those things from yourself. For most women, illness is the only time they take to pay attention to themselves and to grow in self-love. That can only come from taking time for yourself, respecting yourself more, realizing you are deserving of wellness, and loving yourself unconditionally.

3. Regrouping your psychological energy to gain a new perspective on a problem with which you're dealing.

Sometimes a much-needed time out is required to gain objectivity about a pressing situation. It can help you see the issue more clearly, realize where you need to grow and improve, or where you need to change direction. This can also become a time to reflect, realign priorities, reconsider your values, and identify a new purpose for your life.

4. Gaining incentive for personal growth or for modifying undesirable habits.

You may have secretly wanted to make changes in your life but never had the time to think them through. Modified isolation, dropping out for a while, and the peace and quiet that comes with nurturing yourself can provide the time for such personal growth and the time to focus on that challenge. Once a significant disease hits, it is simply easier to quit or modify undesirable habits.

5. Not having to meet your own or others' high expectations.

Although this can seem like a much-needed excuse for nonperformance, it can also be a time when you take back your power. This can be a time when you learn to answer to yourself first, before others, and a time when you become more realistic about your expectations for yourself and your life. It can be a time when you become more forgiving of yourself and of those around you. (70)

In a society where we are so stressed and pushed for time that feelings and emotional needs often take a back seat, disease can fulfill an important purpose. First comes the realization that you needed the time out. Second hopefully comes the gratitude for giving you time to solve the problems in your life, which might have contributed to your disease in the first place.

With illness can come enlightenment and evolve in a more positive way. There are always gifts that illness brings. It's always a matter of perception.

There's got to be a pony in there!

Once there were twin brothers (age five or six) with one being a total pessimist and the other a total optimist. The worried parents took the boys to a psychiatrist since they were concerned the twins had developed extreme personalities.

The doctor treated the young pessimist first. Trying to brighten his outlook, the psychiatrist put the young boy into a room piled to the ceiling with brand-new toys. But instead of being delighted, the little boy burst into tears.

"What's the matter?" the baffled psychiatrist asked. "Don't you want to play with any of the toys?"

"Yes," the little boy bawled, "but if I did, I'd only break them."

Trying to recover from that odd response, the psychiatrist went on to treat the remaining twin, the optimist. In an effort to dampen this little boy's outlook, the psychiatrist took him to a room piled to the ceiling with horse manure. But instead of running away in disgust, the little optimist squealed with delight and clambered to the top of the pile. Dropping to his knees, the youngster began eagerly scooping and scooping with his bare hands.

"What do you think you're doing?" the psychiatrist asked, again as totally baffled as he had been by the first twin.

"With all this manure," the beaming boy replied, "there's got to be a pony in there."

This endearing story reminded me of the chapter on fear and love and how approaches to life can be so different based on our emotional framework at the time. The little pessimist was filled with fear-based emotions as he displayed despair, insecurity, doubt, remorse, dread, distress, apprehension, anxiety, doubt, guilt, panic, and shame. A horrible way to exist.

The little optimist, however, was joyful and expressed love in every aspect of his emotions: joy, delight, confidence, excitement, euphoria, surprise, amazement, expectation, and gratitude. Which set of emotions creates a life that you'd enjoy more?

A one-hundred-year perspective on healing.

I posted in a blog a couple of years ago titled *A 100-Year-Old MD's Perspective on Medicine*, parts of which I thought would be the perfect way to wrap up this book.

A dear friend of mine, Dr. Gladys McGarey, MD, MDH, whom I mentioned earlier, just celebrated her 102nd birthday in November 2022, and she still speaks to groups, is getting ready for a book tour scheduled for 2003, and has a ten-year plan! Are you impressed yet?

I've known Dr. Gladys, as many refer to her, for several decades, and everyone who knows her adores her, especially her past patients. Each of them had the benefit of working with this enlightened medical doctor who was way ahead of her time. She was one of the original cofounders of the AHMA, was instrumental in leading the fight to allow fathers in the delivery room—improving the birthing experiences of women and babies around the world, and helped introduce acupuncture into this country. She has taken impressive action on so many other fronts, too, including in her own practice. She has always been highly intuitive, filled with love, and was born to help people heal. She's loaded with wisdom.

Anyway, I was speaking to the head of her foundation the other day, and Rose Winters shared a quote Dr. Gladys had said recently, which I thought was perfect to share here. This was what she said:

"Medicine is so busy trying to prevent death that it's killing life!"

Dr. Gladys obviously believes in holistic healing, which she has renamed Living Medicine; one I think is equally appropriate. It was from her that I borrowed the earlier comparisons that describe how the tools conventional medicine uses to attack the disease, kill the virus, destroy the bacteria, wipe out parasites, and battle against infection are all tools of warfare. I further explained that doctors are primarily focused on fighting a war against disease and using pharmaceutical drugs as the primary weapon in their arsenal. But as with any war, as she notes as well, there is always collateral damage. The collateral damage is often the side effects of the drugs prescribed, and the victims of that collateral damage are the patients.

Holistic healing, which is also my preferred method of care, works to strengthen the body to do its own fighting. When needed, it employs natural treatments and remedies to help the body shore up its resources to win whatever battle it's engaged.

One method of care, the conventional model, focuses on killing the disease, and the other, the more holistic and natural approach, on healing the body. It's a matter of perspective. I think Dr. Glady's term Living Medicine is wonderful since it's a new way to look at holistic healing; both phrases work for me.

After practicing for seventy years and being a retired centenarian doctor today, my friend, Gladys McGarey, MD, MD(H), always practiced holistic healing first, the more conventional options only if she deemed necessary. Her life exemplifies one's ability to enjoy a vital quality of life right up until the last minute.

A closing story to take us back farther than Dr. Gladys's beginning.

Once upon a time in the seventeenth century, there were individuals in villages whom locals and those from neighboring settlements would seek out for healing. The tools these individuals used were all natural, and the way they applied their gifts was instinctive.

The healer in this story was a woman. She was gifted and was given the title of healer, since men with the same talents were more often referred to as medicine men or something similar. Regardless, this healer was led to a calling that she willingly shared to help those who needed her.

In sharing her gifts, she picked remedies and treatments from nature—since God provided everything she could possibly require—and her eyes were open to recognize each one. Through her amazing gifts and what nature provided, nearly everyone who sought her out benefited and improved.

She was always led to the right answer, and over time remembered and stored various herbs and remedies so they would be on hand immediately. She knew how to set bones, since she could feel bones, muscles, and ligaments in the body, and could sense where other parts of the body were weak or ailing. There was no reference for organs and their function at that time, and it didn't matter. She didn't have to know *why*, she just needed to know *how*.

The beauty of her ability to heal with nature was simple. Within nature is life. That life-force still exists today. Every leaf, every bit of bark, every herb that grows or flower that blossoms is filled with a life-force that brings energy to one experiencing its healing ability. She intuitively knew how to apply those elements and how to instruct her patients to use them later. Of course, they healed because God provided each of those resources.

Today's medicine is much different. It's made from sources no longer alive; chemicals that are man-made, not God made. They have no individual life—no nourishing capability, only the capability to attack something with a fierceness that causes damage in the long run. That is why scientific medicine—or chemically focused medicine—should only be used as a quick solution, to stop acute symptoms until the healing can occur with a life-force that will heal and not kill.

There is wisdom in realizing that pharmaceuticals would be most safely used as the last resort with the preference for routine care coming from healing methods that nurture the body and allow it to heal instead of only attacking the disease without any regard to the effects on the patient later. Medicine's current mission to win at all costs might not always be appropriate. Healers, over the centuries, were more in concert with Dr. Gladys's philosophy and the philosophy surrounding holistic care.

Such a healer as I describe used all the tools at hand, which are still available today, and still might look at today's techniques of surgery, or cutting as their reference then would be, as a methodology that could certainly be warranted, on occasion. Again, in her time, she would not have understood or had decent tools to use such methods effectively, but I'll bet she would have called surgery a Godsend when used in the right hands.

She, and other ancient healers like her, would hope this story might help readers realize that selecting which method to use and when to use it is smart. That using damaging treatments less frequently and only for emergencies is prudent. And using natural healing treatments for more long-term care is wise.

This ancient healer would have said that God intended discretion in caring for our bodies and that He created the medicine of science—not to replace what she or others like her offered—but to augment what they do.

And so, readers of this book, in the end, decided to drop their judgment of methods they might not totally understand, become more open to new and exciting possibilities, and begin honoring the gifts God gave them, which consist of intuition and faith. They also learned to live more in love and less in fear...

... and they lived healthily ever after!

ENDNOTES

1. Adit A. Ginde, Mark C. Liu, Carlos A. Camargo, Jr. "Demographic differences and trends of vitamin D insufficiency in the US population, 1988-2004", Comparative Study-Arch Intern Med. 2009 Mar 23; 169(6):626-32. Dol: 0.1001/arcinternmed.2008.604. *PubMed.ncbi.nlm.nih.gov.*

2. Scott A. Read, Stephanie Obeid, Chantelle Ahlenstiel, Golo Ahlenstiel. "The Role of Zinc in Antiviral Immunity", Adv Nutr.2019 Jl 1;10(4): 696-710.doi:0.1093/advances/nmz014. *Pubmed.ncbi.nim.nih.gov.*

3. Tierney Sneed. "CDC mask mandate for travelers no longer in effect following judge's ruling, official says". CNN Politics on cnn.com

4. Mike Stobbe, AP Medical Writer. "CDC Restates Recommendation for Masks on Planes and Trains" usnews.com. Article by the Associated Press. May 3, 2022.

5. Robby Soave. "CDC No Longer Recommends Social Distancing, Masks in Schools Unless Spread is High" Reason.com August 11, 2022.

6. Published by John Elfein. "COVID-19 deaths reported in the U.S. as of October 5, 2022, by age" Source: https://www.statista.com/statistics/1191568/reported-deaths-from-covid-by-age-us/

7. "When did obesity become a problem?" *Main News Online*, 2022.

8. Gilbert H. Friedell and Isaac Joyner. "The Great Diabetes Epidemic", nwhn.org – *National Women's Health Network.* Mar. 27, 2015.

9. Rabah Kamal and Bradley Sawyer "What do we know about cardiovascular disease spending and outcomes in the United States?" healthsystemtracker.org *KFF.* February 14, 2017.

10. Carrie Macmillan. "What Does It Mean To Be 'Immunocompromised'?" yalemedicine.org – Family Health. May 3, 2022.

11. "History of transplantation". unos.org.

12. T. G. Benedek. "History of the development of corticosteroid therapy". *HIH National Library of Medicine*-national Center for Biotechnology Information. pubmed.ncbi.nim.nih.gov Oct 2021

13. "Worst Pandemics in History. Global Pandemics All-Time List" ADDucation.info.

14. "Anthony Fauci's Net Worth, Career, Biography, Facts, Age, Life Story" from Early Life and Education. Wikibasics.com.

15. Nichole Acevedo. "December was the deadliest, most infectious month since the start of the pandemic." https://www.nbcnews.com/news/us-news/.

16. "Consent for Medical Treatment: Recent Case Law" Enablelaw.com. February 14, 2017.

17. Disclaimer from the VAERS database. *https://vaers.hhs.gov/data.html.*

18. Olivia Cavallaro. "NIH Director Francis Collins Resigns After Documents Reveal Untruths Surrounding Gain-Of-Function Research" *Christianity Daily*. October 6, 2021.

19. Jeffry Tucker. "Dr. Birx Praises Herself While Revealing Ignorance, Treachery, and Deceit" Brownstone Institute. Brownstone.org July 16, 2022.

20. Michael Senger. "Deborah Birx's Guide to Destroying A Country From Within" Brownstone Institute. Brownstone.org July 14, 2022.

21. Kelly Gooch. "California bill aimed at preventing COVID-19 disinformation heads to governor "beckershospitalreview.com – quoting an article in the *New York Times* Tuesday, August 30th, 2022. Confirmation of Governor Newsom signing from CDmedia.com "California Gov. Gavin Newsom Signs Bill Changing Medicine and Proving He Works for BIG PHARMA".

22. James Hill, MD, JD. "Masks can't reduce Covid infection rates or transmission of any virus: Petty" April 18, 2022 (citing testimony quote from "HB1131: Certified Industrial Hygienist Stephen Petty's

Senate Testimony on Why Masks Don't or Can't Work", by Steve Macdonald. *James Hill MD's Newsletter, Substack.* April 2022 also citing "Citizens for Free Speech-A Nation of Defenders" by Denis Rancourt, PhD (July 3, 2020).

23. John Tierney. "Fauci and Walensky Double Down on Failed Covid Response—Lockdowns were oppressive and deadly. But U.S. and WHO officials plan worse for the next pandemic." *Wall Street Journal.* WSJ/OPINION. August 18, 2022.

24. Vanessa Milne. "Should your child wear a mask at school?" *Today's Parent.* April 11, 2022.

25. "FDA authorizes 1st COVID-19 vaccine in United States" *abcnews.com* December 11, 2020.

26. World Council for Health. "Remembering Dr. Vladimir Zelenko: Physician, Scientist, Activist" July 1, 2022.

27. "Ivermectin Prices and Coupons" *WebMDRx.*webmd.com.

28. "Revenue of the worldwide pharmaceutical market from 2001 to 2021 (in billions of US dollars." statista.com. Prices & Access tab Health, *Pharma & Medtech – Pharmaceutical Products & Market.*

29. "Three-year summary for the years ended December 31" *2021 Annual Review.* Pfizer.com.

30. Chris Beyrer. "The Long History of mRNA Vaccines" publichealth.jhu.edu. October 2021.

31. Fact checked by Dana K. Cassell. "Health News: New Study Found 80% of COVID-19 Patients Were Vitamin D Deficient." Healthline.com. October 27, 2020.

32. C. L. Keen, M. E. Gershwin. "Zinc deficiency and immune function" *National Library of Medicine-National Center for Biotechnology Information* NIH pubmed.ncbi.nim.nih.gov.

33. Cleveland Clinic Newsroom. "Can Vitamin C and Zinc Help Fight COVID-19? Recent research shows popular immune health supplements, vitamin C and zinc are no match for COVID-19." 2. 25-21.

34. Wullianallur Raghupathi and Viju Raghupathi. "An Empirical Study of Chronic Diseases in the United States: A Visual Anallytics Approach to Public Health." National Library of Medicine—National

Center for Biotechnology information (NIH). Published online 2018 Mar 1.

35. Joseph Choi. "Fauci: Vaccinated people become 'dead ends' for the coronavirus." Sunday Talk Shows. thehill.com, 5/16/21.

36. Ana Sandoiu. Fact checked by Zia Sherrell, MPH. "How do COVID-19 vaccines compare with other existing vaccines?" *Medical News Today*. December 14, 2020, medicalnewstoday.com.

37. *Centers for Disease Control and Prevention.* "Mumps Vaccination" https://www.cdc.gov/mumps/vaccination.html.

38. Christopher Tremoglie, Commentary Writer. "Dr. Birx's comments about COVID-19 vaccines vindicate Sen. Rand Paul" *Washington Examiner*. July 26, 2022, from the July 29, 2022, issue.

39. "First mRNA vaccine" *Guinness Book of World Records,* Tozinameran COVID-19 vaccine, developed with Pfizer (USA) and eventually approved for use 02 December 2020 in the United States.

40. "When to see a doctor about COVID-19" UCI Health/Orange County CA ucihealth.org April 07, 2020.

41. Dennis Thompson, HealthDay Reporter. "Ventilators: Helping or Harming COVID-19

42. Robert Preidt. "Study: Most N.Y. COVID Patients on Ventilators Died". HealthDay News as reported on WebMD. April 22, 2020, webmd.com.

43. Michelle Rogers. "Fact check: Hospitals get paid more if patients listed as COVID-19, on ventilators" *USA TODAY Network*. Updated April 27, 2020.

44. Robert Redidt, HealthDay Reporter. "Who Says No to Remdesivir as COVID-19 Treatment" *WebMD webmd.com* Nov. 20, 2020.

45. *"Life Expectancy by Country and in the World (2022)" – Worldometer.*

46. Ohlemacher, Stephen. "US Slipping in Life Expectancy Rankings" *Washington Post* (The Associated Press) 12 August 2007. http://www.Washingtonpost.com.

47. Hannah Ritchie. "In which countries do people smoke the most?" *Our World in Data* https://ourworldindata.org/which-countries-smoke-most.

48. "List of countries by traffic-related death rate." *Wikipedia*.

49. Clinically Reviewed by James Gamache. "How Many Prescription Drugs are Prescribed Each Year?" libertybayrecovery.com. August 29, 2022.

50. "Medical Error Statistics" MyMedicalScore.com.

51. Michael Greger, MD, FACLM. "How Much Nutrition Education Do Doctors Get?" NutritionFacts.org Updated, August 30, 2017.

52. Marcia Hams. "Scorecard Shows U.S. Medical Schools Continue to Make Progress in Pharmaceutical Conflict-of-Interest Policies" *COMMUNITY CATALYST. Health Policy Hub.* communitycatalyst. org.

53. Andrew Weil, MD, *Spontaneous Healing* (New York: Alfred A. Knopf, Inc., 1995), pp. 225-226.

54. "Haphazard reporting of deaths in clinical trials: a review of cases of ClinicalTrials.gov records and matched publications—a cross-sectional study" NIH National *Library of Medicine.* 13 Jan 2018.

55. Ethan Huff. "Science" no longer trustworthy: BMJ op-ed suggests all health research should be considered fraudulent until proven otherwise" *NATURAL NEWS* naturalnews.com August 23, 2022.

56. OXFORD ACADEMIC – Clinical Infectious Diseases. *Interpreting Quantitative Cytomegalovirus DNA Testing: Understanding the Laboratory Perspective* – Colleen S. Kraft, Wendy S. Armstrong, Angela M. Caliendo – Journal Article – published 12 March 2012 – under Analytical Test Characteristics.

57. Christiane Northrup, MD, from a promotional flier: "*How to Create a Health Miracle In Your Life*" 1999, p.15.

58. Andrew Weil, MD, *Spontaneous Healing,* (Alfred A. Knopf, Inc.— 1995) pp. 267-269.

59. Andrew Weil, MD, *Spontaneous Healing,* (Alfred A. Knopf, Inc.— 1995) pp. 267-269.

60. Berkeley Lovelace Jr. "FDA expected to authorize new Covid boosters without data from tests in people. The lack of human data means officials likely won't know how much better the new shots are—if at all—until the fall booster campaign is well underway". *NBC News.* August 30, 2022.

61. ProCon.org. "FDA-Approved Prescription Drugs Later Pulled from the Market by the FDA" *Britannica ProCon.org* Last updated on 12/1/2021.

62. Kristina Fiore, Director of Enterprise & Investigative Reporting. – "Want to Know More About mRNA before Your COVID Jab? – A prier on the history, scope and safety of mRNA vaccines and therapeutics." *MedPage Today*, December 3, 2020, medpagetoday.com.

63. Debra Wood, RN. "Average Time Doctors Spend with Patients. What's the Number for Your Physician Specialty?" *staffcare.com*. December 27, 2017.

64. D. B. Larson and S. S. Larson, "Religious Commitment and Health: Valuing the Relationship," Second Opinion: Health, Faith and Ethics 17:1, 1991, 26-40. Larson and Larson's teaching module: "The Forgotten Factor in Physical and Mental Health: What Does the Research Show?" (An Independent Study Seminar: Washington D.C.: National Institute for Healthcare Research 1992).

65. Bernie S. Siegel, MD, *Love Medicine & Miracles,* (New York: Perennial Library, Harper & Row Publishers, 1998), 66.

66. Alan B. Zibluk. Information paraphrased from *The Psychology of Fear*, an article on alanzibluk.com. August 3, 2022.

67. Bernie S. Siegel, MD, *Love Medicine & Miracles*, (New York: Perennial Library, Harper & Row Publishers, 998) 24, 26.

68. (101) Hermina Drah. "Disturbing Stress Statistics & Facts to Check Out in 2022" *distrubmenot.com* Jan 14, 2022.

69. Claire Klobucista. "U.S. Life Expectancy is in Decline. Why Aren't Other Countries Suffering the Same Problem?" COUNCIL ON FOREIGN RELATIONS. cfr.org/in-brief September 8, 2022

70. O. Carl Simonton, MD, Stephanie Matthews-Simonton, and James L. Creighton, Getting Well Again, (New York: Bantam Doubleday Dell Publishing, 1992), 133-134.